YOGAHEALTH

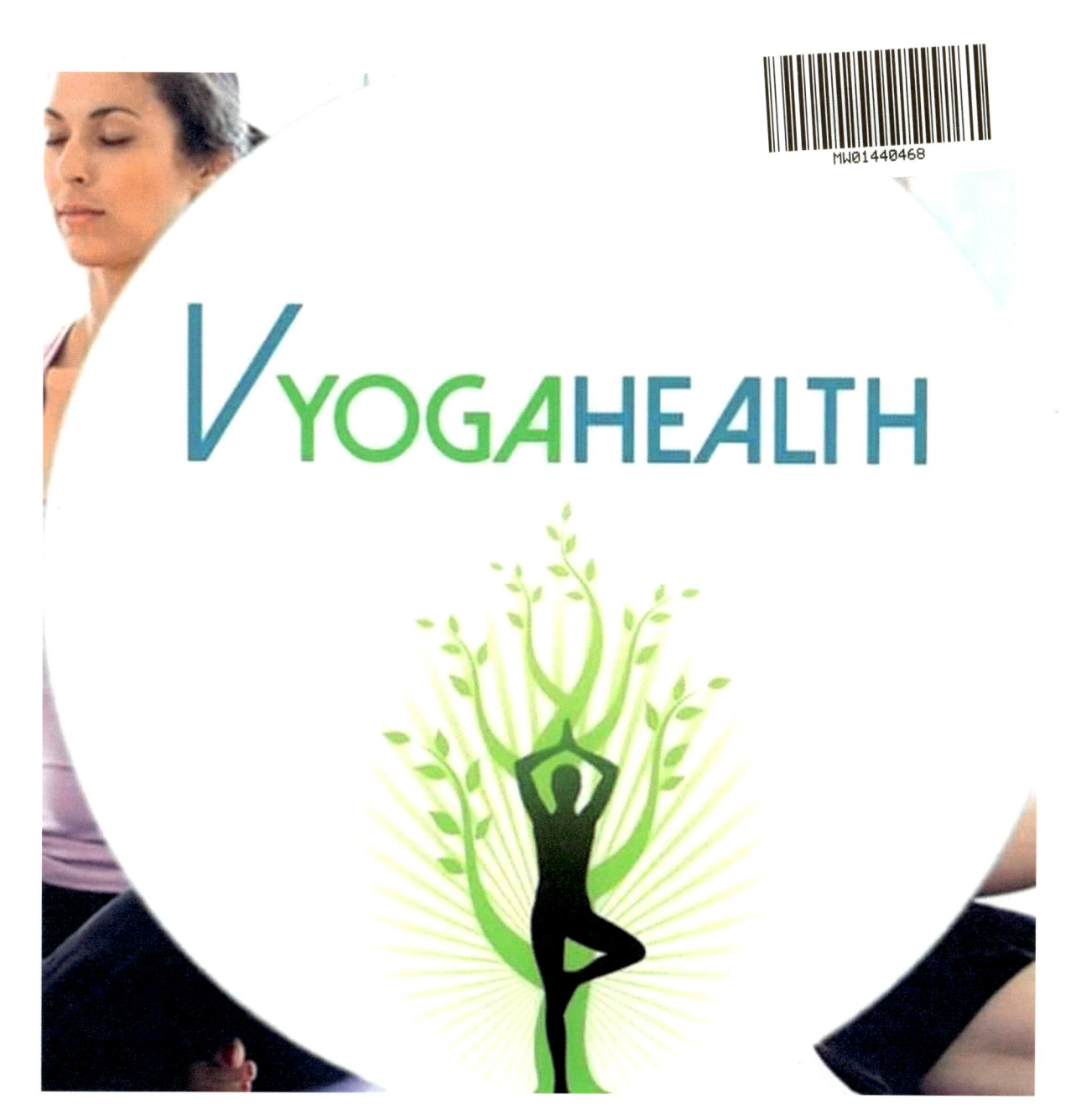

Teacher training RYT200

Enhance Your Knowledge of Yoga

Written by: Veronika Patton

Copyright © 2024 by Veronika Patton

All Rights Reserved

ERYT500

Wellness coach

Educational provider for yoga.

Contact: vyoga4u@gmail.com

Reading Materials

Max Strom A life Worth Breathing.

Light On Yoga By B.K.S Iyengar

Yoga Bible Christina Brown.

The Path To Holistic Health B.K.S Iyengar.

Once the soul awakens the search begins and you can never go back.

From then on, you are consumed with a special longing that will never again let you linger.

Many of us step on the path to spiritual awakening expecting us to lead onward, hoping to become something better than we are and ready to gather all important things.

We need it along the way.

What surprises me is when we eventually realize that this path isn't taking us onward but inward, that we are not gathering things so much as letting them go, and that there was never anything more to aspire to then. The truth of what we already are.

The self - This is an exercise to the self.

I want you to sit down in a quiet room away from everyone.

Take slow steady breaths, inhale through your nose and exhale through the mouth repeat it 5 times.

I want you to take a piece of paper and answer the following questions.

You can email the answers to vyoga4u@gmail.com

The self

- **Who am I?**

This is the biggest and most difficult question for each of us.

- **How will you describe who you are?**

Many people will say about themselves; I am a mother, a nurse, "My name is", and so on. But this is not who we are; we were given those roles by society, by our parents, and so on.

- **Try to define who you are to yourself.**

My favorite quote "I am not this hair, I am not this skin, I am the soul that lives within"

-**By Rumi.**

How do you begin finding the answer to the Question, **"Who am I?"**

I was a person who passed passively through life; I breezed through it as if on autopilot.

I was a passenger just passing through, unable to see through the haze of familiar pain.

It gave me a perspective identity that outlined how I was to view the world and myself.

Fast forward a couple of years, in the midst of a psychological crisis, I decided to embark on a journey toward personal discovery. I set out to establish a purpose, to be sincere, and to tell the truth as best as I can.

This quest involved seeking the answer to one of life's most fundamental questions of human existence:

Who am I, and how do I begin finding the answer to this question?

I thought clues were to be found in the person that I used to be. So, I began gathering the remnants of a deeply fragmented past. I exhumed aspects of life once lived and examined each piece carefully for a thread connecting the past to the present.

I desperately wished to afford my life some semblance of unity and purpose, but the deeper I searched, the more lost I felt. I no longer recognize the person I once knew; she was frigidly unresponsive, beneath heavy layers of cumulative traumas.

I no longer recognized the person that I once was, but this didn't mean that I was lost. I had to shed the layers of an identity that served its purpose at that time but was no longer useful to my present way of being in the world.

Throughout the process of self-discovery, I learned that I could never truly lose myself because the self is anything but a constant and static moment in time.

Finding myself involved in a perpetual phoenix-like state of recapitulation. I found myself realizing that I was never lost to begin with.

So, where do I begin?

"Start with yourself.

Take care of yourself.

Define who you are."

Improve the quality of your actions. " We are what we repeatedly do." Excellence is not an act but a habit.

I aimed to develop great habits through small, tiny actions and micro routines. In doing so, I hoped to maximize the quality of my life in a way that would benefit myself, my friends, my family, and the community.

Examine your fears: "Absolutely everything I need to find is embedded in everything of which I am afraid."

This step was about uncovering what I feared, to recover those repressed elements of the self, into the remainder of my personality.

This involved a conscious effort not to divert my path out of fear; expressed more clearly, if I am on a path and something emerges that frightens me and would compromise the journey forward, I shouldn't avoid it.

The key was to break my fear - past, present, and future - down into manageable, smaller chunks. I devised a strategy of approaches and hopefully, one day in the future, mastery.

I can say wholeheartedly that these steps have been valuable in my journey toward finding the answer to life's most fundamental question of human existence.

They've been a source of comfort and reposed a point on the map when I was feeling wayward and lost. My wish for you is that they become yours, too.

"Just be yourself. "

"We never cease to stand like curious children before the great mystery into which we were born."

-Walter Isaacson.

I am

Humans tend to see things as they aren't.

I am not the person I used to be.

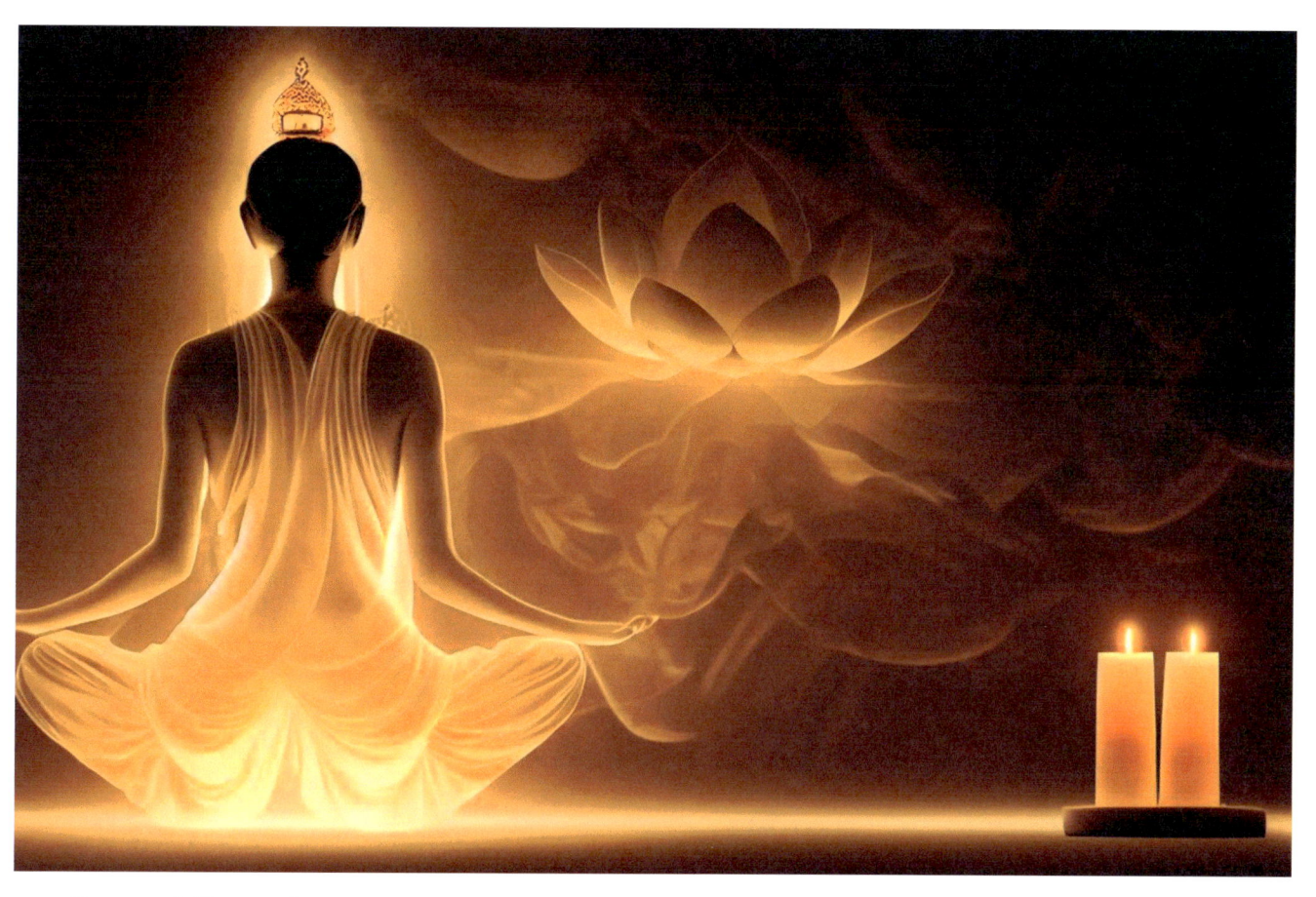

Yoga is different from regular exercise. It goes slow rather than fast.

It emphasizes static postures and fluid rather than rapid motion.

Yoga has a low impact that puts less strain on the body than traditional sports.

Yoga has a minimal approach to burning calories, contracting muscles, and stressing the body's cardiovascular system.

Yoga emphasizes controlling the breath and fostering inner awareness of body position. Yoga draws attention inward.

Yoga can lift moods and resets the body's biological clock.

Yoga in the eyes of a beginner...

Pay attention to the beginner students and modify the positions for them.

- Clarity: Clarity is having the ability to see the mind exactly as it is; to free yourself from judgment, from self-criticism, and from the material world. It's the state of mind that simply knows to let yourself exist here and now.
- Notice your breath: Notice how the air fills your lungs and expands into your belly. Notice the cycle of breath; without breath, we have no life. Calm your mind and relax your body. Being happy every day is a gift.
- Teacher: As the teacher you join the room, take a seat, and absorb the energy of the room around you. You are in charge of creative, positive energy; it is your job to lead the class.
- Get familiar with simple, basic sequences.
- Maintain your own yoga practice by attending other classes.
- Remember the sequences.
- Savasana (corpse pose) rejuvenates the students after a long class. It seals the class.
- One hour of class - Savasana can be 5 min.
- 90 min. class - Savasana can be 10 min.
- Savasana is an asana. It is the time to rest, or close with seated meditation.

Skills to train a private class:

- Ability to bond privately with your student.
- Create trust, patience, connections, self-awareness, and curiosity.
- Learn the ability to engage with the whole person.
- Be present.
- Build strong relationships even when you are busy meeting students where they are.
- Provide what they need on a physical and emotional level and challenge them in a way that makes sense for them.

Teaching Yoga to a Group

- Be present. Teach your students tools and recreate the experience.
- Find out each student's goals and work with them on their goals.
- Class should be a workout - emotionally, spiritually, and energetically calming.
- Create awareness of the physical body.
- Give students more challenging and interesting asanas.
- Help your students ground and calm by connecting with their breathing.
- Focus on the breath.
- You need students to trust you.

- Always show up on time.
- Be professional.
- Continuously learn and grow in your knowledge.
- Have students share things and never share them with anyone else.

Difficult clients

- Always late.
- Canceling.
- Disinterested.
- Not listening when being instructed.
- Unfriendly.

Stand confidently in the power of a teacher.

- Don't let them get to you; it's not about you.
- Even if they are difficult students, love your students.
- Show up with clarity, warmth, confidence, and consistency. Keep showing up.
- Always deeply believe that transformation can and will happen
- Feel deep compassion for all of your clients.
- Know that if someone behaves badly, it is from a place of pain.
- Be clear about boundaries, and consistently enforce them.

I want you to do one exercise

What does Yoga mean to you?

Please email it to vyoga4u@gmail.com

Please learn the entire sequence below!

Yoga sequence for class: Please memorize it. You will have to record yourself doing these sequences.

Integration

- Exhale Child's Pose
- Exhale Down Dog
- Exhale Rag Doll
- Inhale Halfway Lift
- Exhale Forward Fold

Sun Salutation A

- Inhale Mountain Pose - Arms Up
- Exhale Hands to Heart
- Inhale Mountain Pose - Arms Up
- Exhale Forward Fold
- Inhale Halfway Lift
- Exhale Chaturanga
- Inhale Up Dog

Sun Salutation B

- Chair pose - inhale
- Forward Fold - exhale
- Halfway Lift - inhale
- Chaturanga - exhale
- Upward Facing Dog - inhale
- Downward Facing Dog - exhale
- Right side Warrior 1 - inhale
- Chaturanga - exhale
- Upward Facing Dog - inhale
- Downward Facing Dog - exhale
- Left Side Warrior 1 - inhale
- Chaturanga - exhale
- Upward Facing Dog - inhale
- Downward Facing Dog – exhale

Sun Salutation B - Variation

- Chair pose - inhale
- Forward Fold - exhale
- Halfway Lift - inhale
- Chaturanga - exhale
- Upward Facing Dog - inhale
- Downward Facing Dog - exhale
- Right side Warrior 1 - inhale
- Warrior 2 - exhale
- Reverse Warrior - inhale
- Chaturanga - exhale
- Upward Facing Dog - inhale
- Downward Facing Dog - exhale
- Left Side Warrior 1 - inhale
- Warrior 2 - exhale
- Reverse Warrior - inhale
- Chaturanga - exhale
- Upward Facing Dog - inhale
- Downward Facing Dog - exhale
- Raise your right leg high
- Bend your knee, stack your hips
- Flip dog knee, stack your hips
- Flip dog or wild thing
- Flip back to three-legged dog
- Crescent lunge - inhale
- Hands to heart - exhale
- Inhale - Lengthen your spine forward
- Exhale - twist right
- inhale - lengthen
- Exhale - twist
- Inhale - open your arms floor to ceiling
- Exhale - warrior 2
- Inhale - reverse warrior
- Exhale - side angle lunge
- Inhale - reverse warrior
- Exhale - chaturanga

- Inhale - upward-facing dog
- Exhale - downward facing dog

REPEAT ON THE LEFT SIDE

- Travel to the top of your mat
- Inhale - halfway lift
- Exhale - forward fold
- Inhale - chair pose
- Exhale - hands to heart
- Take a breath in
- Twist right - exhale
- Inhale - lengthen.
- Exhale - twist
- Inhale - arms floor-to-ceiling
- Exhale forward fold
- Split your feet and hips a distance apart
- Grab your big toes with your peace fingers (or first 2 fingers)
- Inhale - halfway lift
- Exhale - fold

REPEAT ON THE LEFT SIDE
*** You will stand on your palms in a forward fold instead***

- Crow poses or malasana (Garland pose or deep squat)
- Chaturanga
- Inhale - upward-facing dog
- Exhale - downward facing dog
- Right foot forward crescent lunge (high lunge)
- Left arm under, right arm over - eagle arms
- Left leg over right - eagle
- Inhale mountain pose
- Exhale hands to heart
- Right foot up - dancers pose
- Slowly release
- Inhale arms
- Exhale fold forward
- Inhale halfway fit
- Chaturanga

- Up dog
- Down dog
- Left foot forward - crescent lunge
- Right arm under, left arm over - eagle arms
- Right leftover left - eagle
- Inhale mountain pose
- Exhale hands to heart
- Left foot up - dancers pose
- Slowly release - hands to heart
- Tree pose - right foot up
- Release
- Tree pose - left foot up
- Release - hands to heart
- Inhale mountain pose
- Exhale forward fold
- Inhale halfway lift
- Chaturanga
- Up dog
- Down dog

Triangle Series

- Right side - Warrior 1
- Warrior 2
- Reverse triangle
- Triangle
- Rise to stand
- Wide-legged forward fold
- Rise up
- Warrior 2
- Reverse Warrior
- Chaturanga
- Up dog
- Down dog

Repeat Left side

Backbends/Abs

- From Downward-facing dog
- Inhale - shift forward to plank
- Exhale - slowly lower your belly
- Locust pose - 2 or 3 rounds with different variations
- Floor bow

**In these belly backbends you lift on the inhale and lower on the exhale; for floor bow, you would say, "Inhale, lift up, kick back…etc." **

Place your hands under your shoulders and press yourself up so that you are standing on your knees.

- Camel pose
- Slowly rise up
- Down dog with bent knees - sweep your hips from side to side
- Camel pose
- Slowly rise up
- Sit back on heels
- Shift your hips to the right and come into navasana (Boat Pose).
- Hold in navasana - 5 breaths
- Lower down halfway
- Lift up 5x
- Lower all the way to the ground.
- Set up for bridge pose.
- Lift your hips (for 5 breaths)
- Slowly lower down.

**Can start to alternate core with backbends - bridge or full wheel Supta baddha konasana (Reclining Bound Angle Pose). **

The Business of Yoga

- You will be an independent contractor
- You will need Yoga insurance coverage from Yoga Alliance.
- Be professional at all times.
- Create a resume and keep it up to date with a short bio about yourself.
- You will need teacher certification.
- Create a class including a style transition for the class.
- Set an intention and focus on your intention.
- If you start in a studio, you might want to start volunteering and offer your help, like cleaning after some classes.
- Go to workshops and be consistent with your knowledge and practice.
- There are many Yoga teachers. You need to be persistent and have your own style.

How do we manage our energy and time as teachers?

- Having clear boundaries in a relationship between you and your students.
- Create the structure and safety of meaningful work.
- Be clear on your boundaries regarding time and money. This is the first step in creating a safe container.
- This means keeping a consistent schedule and having a clear 24- hour cancellation policy.
- Your teaching space should be separate from your money space.
- Handle all payments and scheduling via email.
- Don't share your stories or anything private. You are at work.
- Don't share personal, heartfelt boundaries unless they resonate with the students.
- Take care of yourself, and be clear with your boundaries, time, and money.
- Be clear about how you organize your schedule.
- Make time for your own practice and caring for yourself.

"We can't take care of other people if you are not taking care of yourself. "

1. Your energetic space is deeply present.
2. Feel the vibe in the room and take charge as the leader and teacher in charge. Your goal is to assist your students to feel better than when they came in.
3. Things to do to connect with students:
    - Smile.
    - Exercise with your students.
    - Make eye contact with every student.

- Model proper breath techniques with students
- Modify postures for each level of students.
- At the beginning of the class, ask the students if there is an area on which they would like to work.
- Encourage, motivate, acknowledge and support students through the journey and practice of Yoga.

"Mind the Gap"

Understanding the nature of the human mind through yoga philosophy reminds us to pay attention to the space between where we are standing and where we want to go.

The value gap is the space between our professed values versus what we do, think and feel. Part of it is also spiritual values.

"Strategy"

The game plan of the detailed answer to the question "What is my business strategy?" In any profession, we should have a game plan of the goals we want to accomplish.

"Culture"

The definition of what we want to achieve is determined by who we are and our surroundings.

If we want to isolate the problem and develop information strategies, we have to hold our aspirational values up against what we call our practical values. It is how we actually feel, behave, and think.

"Disengagement "

Disengagement is the result of leaders not living by the same values they preach.

"We can't give people what we don't have. Who we are matters immeasurably more than what we know, or who we want to be."

"Aspirational values"

- Honesty and integrity versus letting things slide.
  For example – a mom goes to the grocery store with her children and the cashier forgets to charge her for the soda. She doesn't return the soda.
- Respect and accountability are of paramount importance.
- Gratitude and respect. Don't take people for granted and disrespect others. For example - if both parents are yelling at each other in front of the child, the child will also become agitated and act out or cry.
- Setting boundaries and limits. For example- a parent has to set limits for their teenagers because they often lack the self-control and wisdom to make good choices.

- Emotional connection and honored feelings. For example, discussing and sharing experiences that were hard in the past will often inform the child's life in the future.

The lesson that we must learn in our lives is to mind the gap. We must pay close attention to the space between where we are standing, and where we want to be. If we want to teach our children honesty, we must model that behavior.

Leadership

Being a leader doesn't give us the right to insult others.

Being a leader is an example for others. Leaders should have the courage to be vulnerable, to take responsibility, and to take risks. Leaders should be able to resonate with other people.

There is no winning. Not everyone can take the discomfort of leadership. Leadership is learning to be uncomfortable at times. Leadership requires us to move from our comfort zone to reach our full potential.

As leaders, we must create a vision while teaching yoga and live up to that.

"There is no vision without visibility."

PNF stretching: Stretching, tensing, and relaxing

PNF is a stretching technique that increases ROM (range of motion) and flexibility.

PNF increases ROM by increasing the length of the muscle and increasing neuromuscular efficiency.

PNF stretching has been found to increase ROM in trained and untrained individuals.

Facts about Flexibility

- Many people are not flexible, so they don't practice.
- There should be a fine line between being uncomfortable and having pain.
- Females are more flexible than males due to their bone structure.
- Breath creates heat in the body.

PNF HAMSTRING AND GLUTEAL STRETCH

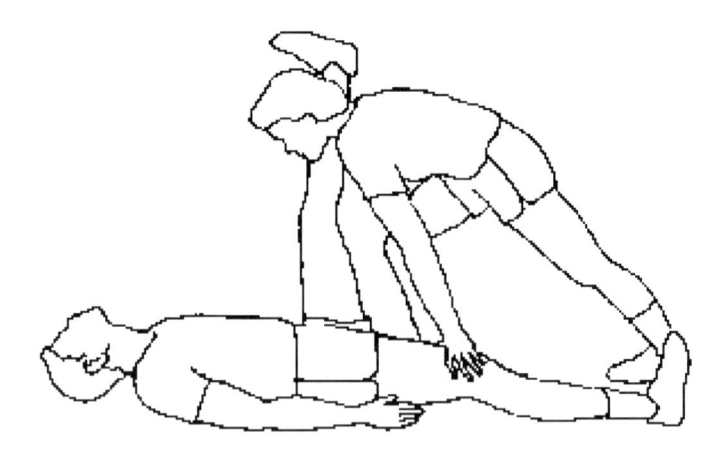

PNF CHEST STRETCH

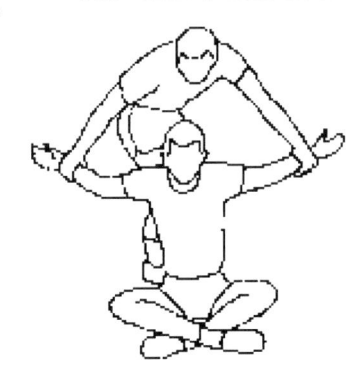

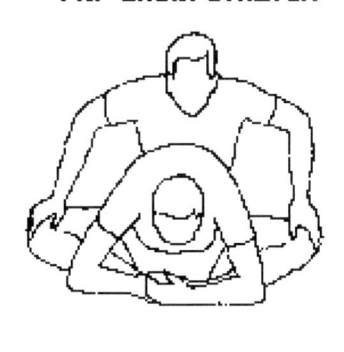

PNF GROIN STRETCH

Reference: AR 350-15 Army Physical Fitness Program. November 1989.

Static posture

Static posture is when a person is standing, sitting, or lying still. So, a static pose for your superhero is one where the character is standing, sitting, or lying still.

Dynamic stretching

Dynamic stretching is a movement-based type of stretching.

It uses the muscles themselves to bring about a stretch. It's different from traditional "static" stretching because the stretch position is not held.

Ballistic stretching

Ballistic stretching uses the momentum of a moving body or a limb to force it beyond its normal range of motion. This is stretching by bouncing into, or out of, a stretched position.

This technique uses the stretched muscles as a spring to pull you out of the stretched position.

Bandhas in yoga are energy locks or binds meant to tighten or close off areas of the body. Western practitioners may also refer to bandhas as energetic locks or seals.

Mula bandha

Like asana practice, mula bandha is intended to purify the pranamayakosha—one of the subtle, five-layered sheaths of the energetic body. On the pranic level, mula bandha redirects the energy of apana, the aspect of prana within the body that naturally flows downward from the navel.

Uddiyana Bandha

Uddiyana bandha is considered one of the three classical bandha asanas. Not only is it practiced to strengthen and tone abdominal muscles, but also to practice meditative, controlled breathing and to energize the body. In Sanskrit, uddiyana means "upward" and bandha means "binding," "uniting" or "contracting.

- Feel supported first; seated and comfortable.
- First, empty the lungs & belly by controlled exhalation.
- When the lungs & belly are completely empty, suck the navel in and up.
- Now, hold your breath and the abdomen gently for 8 to 12 counts.
- Release the abdomen and breathe out.

To enter the pose, begin in a standing position on the mat with feet set apart the distance of the hips. Slightly angle the body forward from the waist and bend the knees lightly. Ground the hands on the knees or tops of the thighs. Take a deep inhalation while pushing the stomach forward, then forcefully and quickly exhale until the lungs are completely empty. Tighten the abs until the navel area is pulled back against the mid-spine. Hold the pose until the next inhalation (about five to 15 seconds) and repeat three to 10 rounds of this abdominal lock.

Uddiyana bandha is known as upward abdominal lock in English.

Uddiyana bandha from a standing or seated position. It is recommended for beginners to practice it in a standing position before attempting the asana from a comfortable seated position on the mat for Pranayama.

In a spiritual yoga practice, it is believed that one should not do an **uddiyana bandha** without a **mula bandha**. It is thought that **uddiyana bandha** completes the mula bandha, as the **uddiyana bandha** continues to move energy harnessed through the chakras to the heart with more force than practicing the **mula bandha** alone.

Mudras are a set of subtle physical movements that can change one's mood, attitude, or perspective, which helps to increase concentration and alertness.

A **mudra** can be a simple hand position, or it can encompass the entire body in a combination of **Asana**, **Pranayama**, **Bandha**, and visualization methods.

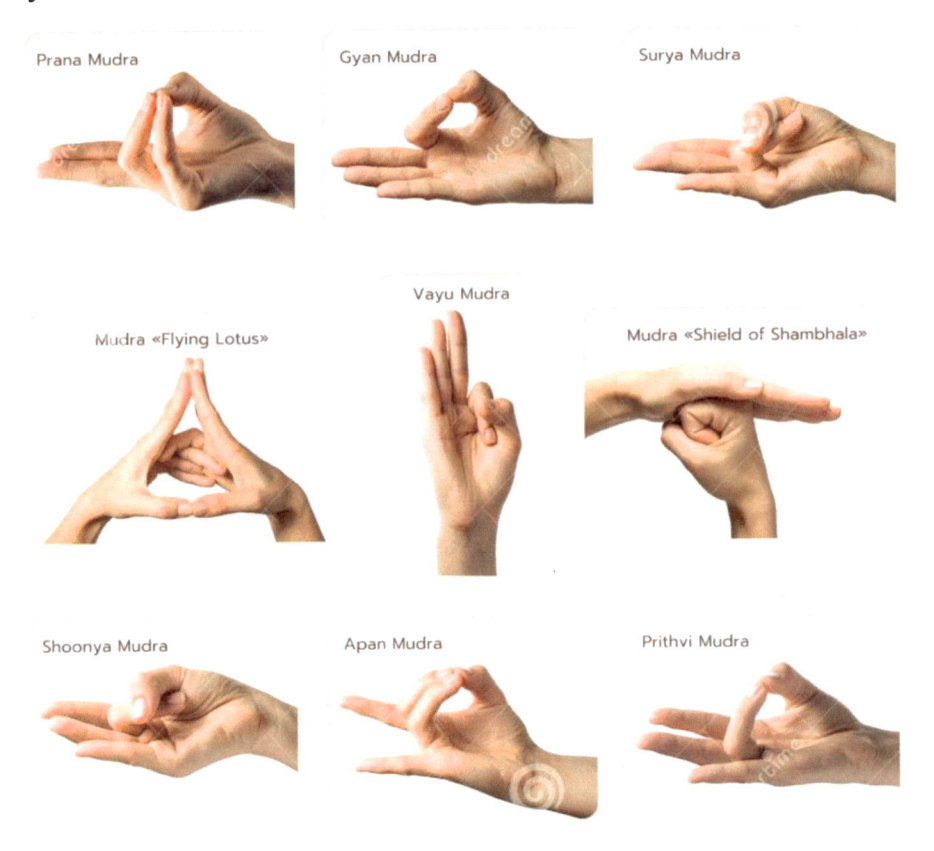

Cueing for down-facing dog pose

While students are in down-facing dog, you can have them bend one knee at a time, followed by a breath. Another variation: with inhales rise on your toes, and with exhales lower your heels to the mat.

From down-facing dog to the front of the mat. Float or walk to the front of the mat

- Bring feet to legs
- Lift your heels and bend your knees
- Rise to your toes
- Spring to the front of your mat
- Breath
- Pay attention to your breath and you will feel healthier and more alert.
- Breathing deeply widens the lung capacity.

Balloon breathing

Inhaling through the nose, expanding the belly like a balloon while exhaling through the nose.

Imagine a balloon inside of you. Imagine filling the balloon with one arm on the belly and the other on the chest. Bring your awareness to your breath and notice how the stomach and chest rise with each inhale

As you breathe out and exhale, imagine the balloon slowly emptying and falling gently into your stomach.

- Breathe through your nose.
- Relax all your facial muscles.
- Try to make each exhalation and inhalation even.
- Breathe as deeply as you can, but don't hold your breath.
- Focus on your breath.

Breathing exercises

When you breathe deeply, imagine that all the good things in your life, happiness, and space are flowing into your body with each breath. As you breathe out imagine that negativity is flowing out.

Different meanings

"**Yoga**" is a Sanskrit word meaning to yoke, to join, or to unite. The practice of yoga aims to unite the body, mind, and spirit as well as personal and Universal awareness.

Just as a yoke is a mechanism of control and unity, yogic practice is a mechanism of controlling the body, breath, senses and mind to enable more effective meditation for the purpose of liberation.

Parana in Sanskrit means the ancient Indian language from which the word "yoga" was born"prana" translates to "vital energy" or "life force."

The Vedas, a collection of revered ancient Hindu texts, teach that yogis must increase and conserve prana through lifestyle choices, balancing it through yoga, meditation, and diet.

The Five Elements of Yoga – The five elements are **Prithvi** (earth), **Jal** (water), **Agni** (fire), **Vayu** (air), and **Akasha** (ether or space.) **Ayurveda**, the sister science of yoga and one of the oldest medical systems is still practiced today.

Tapas is derived from the Sanskrit root "tap," which means to heat or to burn. In yoga, it refers to the practice of self-discipline, self-control, perseverance, and austerity. The ancient yogis discovered that a fiery passion is necessary for spiritual awakening and transformation.

Asana is a Sanskrit word meaning "posture," "seat," or "place." Asanas are the physical positions we assume during a hatha yoga practice.

Ashtanga Yoga: The word **Ashtanga** is composed of two Sanskrit words, "Ashta" and "Anga." "Ashta" refers to the number eight, while "Anga" means limb or body part. Therefore, **Ashtanga** is the union of the eight limbs of yoga into one complete, holistic system.

8 Limbs of Yoga

1. YAMA – Restraints, moral disciplines or moral vows
2. NIYAMA – Positive duties or observances
3. ASANA – Posture
4. PRANAYAMA – Breathing Techniques
5. PRATYAHARA – Sense withdrawal
6. DHARANA – Focused Concentration
7. DHYANA – Meditative Absorption
8. SAMADHI – Bliss or Enlightenment

Bhagavad Gita means "song." Religious leaders and scholars interpret the word Bhagavad in several ways. Accordingly, the title has been interpreted as "the word of God" by the theistic schools, "the words of the Lord," "the Divine Song," and "Celestial Song" by others.

Ma Jaya Sati Bhagavati

Ma Jaya Sati Bhagavati is an American-born spiritual teacher who is widely known for her work serving the homeless, the poor, and people living with AIDS.

She is also a gay activist and a forerunner in the struggle for human rights and religious freedom, participating in interfaith and inter-religious dialogues and dedicating her life to peace.

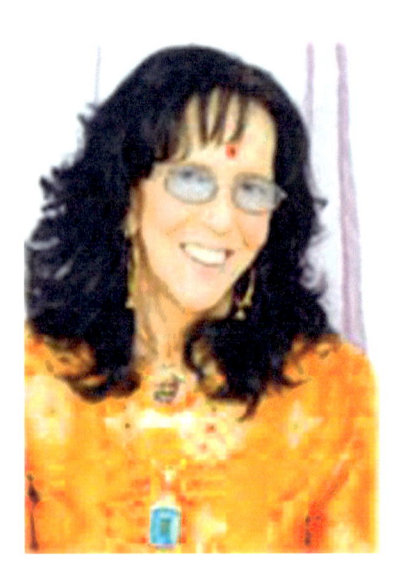

Ma Jaya Sati Bhagavati

Ma Jaya grew up in poverty and was homeless for years, an experience which she credits with teaching her to respect the dignity of every human being.

In 1972, she underwent a powerful spiritual awakening in which she felt the presence of Christ. Later, she met her teacher, the great Indian saint Swami Nityananda, whose influence formed the basis of her teaching.

In 1976, Ma Jaya established in Florida, the Kashi Foundation and Ashram, an interfaith residential community and teaching center also known as Neem Karoli Baba Kashi Ashram.

She has since established centers in New York, Los Angeles, Washington, D.C., Santa Fe, Chicago, Atlanta and London. She also serves as a trustee on the Governing Council of the Parliament of the World's Religions.

In 1990, Ma Jaya founded the River Fund as a service arm of the Kashi Foundation. The River Fund also helps fund impoverished townships in Cape Town, South Africa. In addition, Ma's fund supports the Providence Orphanage in Uganda, orphanages in Mexico, and AIDs Treatment Access Programs in Cuba and South Africa. In 1997, supported by the Dalai Lama, she founded World Tibet Day.

Ma's teachings are founded in Hindu philosophy and integrate many faith traditions. As a Master of **Kundalini Yoga**, Ma created the path of **Kali Yoga**, the yoga of the Mother, which accesses the energy of the Divine Mother. Her teachings focus on attaining spiritual fulfillment through selfless service to humanity.

Bhakti- (Sanskrit: भक्ति) means "attachment, participation, fondness for, homage, faith, love, devotion, worship, purity." It was originally used in Hinduism, referring to devotion and love for a personal god or a representational god by a devotee.

The Yamas and Nimas – The five yamas (social ethics) and five niyamas (personal observances) are two of the eight limbs of yoga. The Yamas are **Ahimsa** (nonviolence), **Satya** (truthfulness), **Asteya** (non-stealing), **Brahmacharya** (abstinence), and **Aparigraha** (non-accumulation). The yamas primarily guide our actions when we interact with others.

The five niyamas - **Soucha** (internal and external cleanliness), **Santosha** (being happy and content), **Tapas** (penance), **Swadhyaya** (self-study) and **Ishvarapranidhana** (surrender to the higher power) are focused on the practitioner's physical and psychological well-being.

As a yoga teacher you should highlight the yamas and nimas to illustrate that a yoga practice is not restricted to sessions on a rectangular mat. These principles allow students of yoga to carry their practice into their daily lives.

Bikram yoga is a type of hot yoga in which practitioners perform 26 asanas (poses) and two Pranayama breathing exercises in a room heated to at least 104 degrees Fahrenheit.

The Bikram method is the original hot yoga practice, invented in the 1970s by yoga teacher Bikram Choudhury.

Indra Devi, the daughter of European nobility who introduced the ancient discipline of yoga to the Kremlin leadership, Hollywood stars like Gloria Swanson and even students in India, died in Buenos Aires at the age of 102. In Buenos Aires, where she had lived for several years, she formed a yoga foundation that was named after her.

Known to her followers as **Mataji**, which means mother, she was a student of Sri Tirumalai Krishnamacharya, the legendary guru who gained worldwide attention for stopping his heartbeat for two minutes. At a time when yoga was almost an exclusively masculine pursuit, she was his first female student.

Two of his other students, B.K.S. Ayengar and K. Pattabhi Jois, both men, took his essential teachings and built a style of yoga accessible to Westerners, characterized by gentleness.

Guru (/ˈɡuːruː/ Sanskrit: गुरु, IAST: guru; Pali: garu) is a Sanskrit term for a "mentor, guide, expert, or master" of certain knowledge or field.

Guru is used in a similar way as Sherpa to refer to someone good at something or an expert in a subject matter. The word guru, however, comes from Buddhist and Hindu religions and refers to a spiritual guide or leader held in high esteem.

The practice of **Hatha yoga** aims to join, yoke, or balance these two energies. A yoga class described as 'Hatha' will typically involve a set of physical postures (yoga poses) and breathing techniques. These are typically practiced more slowly and with more static posture holds than a **Vinyasa flow** or **Ashtanga class**.

Shoulder Stand, also known as **Salamba Sarvangasana** in some yoga traditions, is a challenging introductory pose.

The pose is an inversion, meaning you are upside down. It creates health benefits for your back, heart, and digestive system.

B.K.S. Iyengar yoga is "meditation in action." His teaching combines all eight elements in asana practice, which helps us explore and experience the rest. This brings us back into contact with the outside world, awakened by the basic understanding that everything and everyone is interconnected.

Jnana is Sanskrit for "knowledge or wisdom," and **Jnana Yoga** is the path of attaining knowledge of the true nature of reality through meditation, self-inquiry, and contemplation.

The word "**Karma**" means action, so **Karma Yoga** is the Yoga of Action or duty. **Karma Yoga** is defined as: "Doing your duty at your best without any involvement of ego or attachment." In this definition of **Karma Yoga**, there are four essential words: duty, ego, attachment, and expectation of reward.

Its purpose is to activate your **Kundalini energy** or **Shakti**. This is a spiritual energy that's said to be located at the base of your spine. As **Kundalini yoga** awakens this energy, it's supposed to enhance your awareness and help you move past your ego. Sometimes, the practice is also called "yoga of awareness."

A mantra is a motivating chant, like the "I think I can, I think I can" you repeat to yourself on the last stretch of a race. A mantra is usually a repeated word or phrase, but it can also refer more specifically to a word repeated in meditation.

Meditation, which is the practice of focused concentration, entails bringing yourself back to the moment. Meditation manages stress, whether positive or negative. Meditation can also reduce areas of anxiety, chronic pain, depression, heart disease, and high blood pressure.

Om or aum (pronounced ah-uu-mm) is a sacred sound considered by many ancient philosophical texts to be the sound of the universe, encompassing all other sounds within it. In Sanskrit, om is called Pranava, which means to hum and is considered an unlimited or eternal sound.

Who was Patanjali?

Patanjali was a sage in India who is believed to have authored several Sanskrit works, the most prominent of which is the Yoga Sutras, a classical yoga text dating to 200 BCE – 200 CE. Though references to yoga within Hindu scripture had already long existed, it's believed they were too diverse and complex for the general public, so Patanjali created the Yoga Sutras to compile existing teachings into a format that is easier to understand and follow.

Today, the Yoga Sutras are the most commonly referenced text on yoga, making Patanjali "the father of yoga" in the eyes of many. Beyond the Yoga Sutras, commentaries on two other notable works are attributed to Patanjali as well. One of them is the Mahabhashya, dating from about the second century BCE, is a commentary on an authoritative Sanskrit grammar text written by the Indian grammarian Panini. The other is the Carakavarttika, dating somewhere between the eighth and 10th centuries, which is a commentary on the Charaka Samhita, a large treatise on Ayurveda (traditional Indian) medicine.

While modern scholars believe this timeline makes it impossible for it to have been the same Patanjali who compiled all three of these works, many scholars hold a more traditional view that a single Patanjali is indeed responsible for all three. Some might think it ridiculous for anyone to believe that a single person could be the author of texts written possibly more than 1,000 years apart. However, Patanjali is also considered by many within the Hindu tradition to be a divine figure.

As written by David Gordon White in his book "The Yoga Sutra of Patanjali: A Biography," "'Patanjali' is listed as the name of one of the 26 mythical divine serpents in a number of Puranas." The major Puranas (18 in number) are ancient Hindu texts said to have been composed by the sage **Veda Vyasa**. The Vishnudharmottara Purana, a supplement to the Vishnu Purana, says the "image of Patanjali's Yoga teaching should have the form of Ananta." Ananta is described in Hindu legend to be the divine Lord of Serpents who is said to hold all of the planets of the universe on his 1,000 cobra hoods.

The Vishnudharmottara Purana, which dates to the sixth century, makes a connection between the "Yoga' Patanjali and the "Ananta" Patanjali, as if they are the same. Taking note of this, King Bhoja — an 11th-century patron of arts, literature, and science — wrote in the introduction of his "Royal Sun" commentary of Patanjali's Yoga Sutras: "I bow with folded hands to Patanjali, the best of sages, who removed the impurities of the mind through yoga; the impurities of speech through grammar; and the impurities of the body through medicine. To he whose upper body has a human form, who holds a conch and a wheel, who is white and has a thousand heads, to that Patanjali, I offer obeisance."

King Bhoja's praise of Patanjali not only recognizes the "Yoga" and "Ananta" Patanjali to be the same person but also the "Grammar" and "Ayurveda" Patanjali. Though there are other instances of the four-in-one Patanjali portrayal throughout history Bhoja's prayer has become one of the more well-known and recited examples. Of the three works, the Yoga Sutras have been especially influential on modern culture."

The first two parts of Patanjali's process are **Yama** (restraint from unethical actions) and **Niyama** (observance of positive actions), which help to control the lower instincts of one's nature and cultivate good character. The next three, asana (physical postures), **Pranayama** (breath control), and **Pratyahara** (sense withdrawal), enable control over the body, breath, and senses. Finally, **Dharana** (concentration) and **Dhyana** (meditation), help one to control the mind, leading the yogi to **Samadhi** (absorption with the Divine).

This system is known as **Ashtanga yoga** (literally "eight limbs") — not to be confused with capital-a Ashtanga yoga, which is a specific method of yoga practice taught by the late K Pattabhi Jois and other teachers following in his lineage. The Bhagavad Gita, probably the best-known religious text of Hinduism, states that liberation is attained with the help of the mind. It also states that the mind is the best of friends for one who has conquered it, but the greatest enemy to one who fails to do so.

Although the process outlined in the Yoga Sutras does indeed help to instill relaxation and physical health — the contemporary multi-billion dollar yoga industry focuses nearly exclusively on this — yoga is more accurately a process of controlling the mind in pursuit of liberation. Though we may never know the full truth of Patajali's life (or lives) to the standards of modern academic historians, the fact remains that a huge number of people have been and continue to be inspired and uplifted by the practice of yoga. Regardless of the dates of origin or whether authored by one or several, the influence of these texts has continued to affect and transform the lives of millions.

Guru Goraknath

In his Goraksha-Shatakam , Guru Goraknath does not use the terms of Hatha Yoga or Raja Yoga nor the Ashtanga Yoga terminology of Patanjali. The term he uses is Shadanga Yoga, referring to a Yoga of six limbs, with the implication that Yama and Niyama have already been learned and internalized The six limbs are Asana (bodily postures), Pranayama (breath control), Pratyahara (composure), Dharana (concentration), Dhyana (immersion) and Samadhi (union). In Hindu yoga, samadhi is the highest of the eight limbs of yoga. Samadhi is the experience of spiritual enlightenment when the self, the mind, and the object of meditation merge into one (union).

Swami Rama

Swami Rama became famous for his ability to control his body in yoga nidra, writing many books, including the autobiographical Living with Himalayan Masters.

Ramakrishna Paramahansa

Ramakrishna Paramahansa, also spelled Ramakrishna Paramahamsa, born Gadadhar Chattopadhay or Chatterjee, was an Indian Hindu mystic and spiritual leader. He was a popular teacher, speaking in rustic Bengali with stories and parables. Ramakrishna's main teachings included God's realization as the supreme goal of life, renunciation of Kama-Kanchana, Harmony of Religions and Jiva is Shiva.

Sage - As opposed to a philosopher, the sage (or "sophos") in ancient Greece was considered the bearer of wisdom: someone who already possessed wisdom and only needed to self-actualize himself.

Samadhi - a state of intense concentration achieved through meditation. In Hindu yoga, this is regarded as the final stage, at which union with the divine is reached (before or at death).

On a very basic level, they look like this

- Yamas: external disciplines, like universal values.
- Niyama: internal disciplines, like personal observation.
- Asana: poses or postures.
- Pranayama: breath control.
- Pratyahara: withdrawal of the senses.
- Dharana: concentration.
- Dhyana: meditation.
- Samadhi: bliss, or union.

Sanskrit: Sanskrit is the sacred language of Hinduism, the language of classical Hindu philosophy, and of historical texts of Buddhism and Jainism.

Soma - The Hindu sun god represents sun and light.

Tantra Yoga - Tantra is a type of yoga that weaves together many different techniques, such as mantra meditation, visualization, mudras, Pranayama, and initiation to study the inner universe through our human body. These Tantric techniques and rituals primarily focus on the cultivation and build-up of kundalini energy.

ViniYoga - ViniYoga is a comprehensive and authentic transmission of the teachings of yoga, including āsana, prāṇāyāma, bandha, sound, chanting, meditation, personal ritual and study of texts. Viniyoga (prefixes vi and ni plus yoga) is an ancient Sanskrit term that implies **differentiation, adaptation**, and **appropriate application**.

Visualization Practise - Visualization is a style of meditation where the practitioner focuses their attention on a positive image, thought, feeling, or sensation. In this type of meditation, the practitioner will visualize an image or concept in their mind's eye and remain focused on this image during the practice.

Yoga - Yoga is a Sanskrit word which means union. The literal meaning is "to yoke". The word Yoga is derived from the Sanskrit root word "yuj," which means to join, to integrate, or to harness. A Hindu spiritual and ascetic discipline, a part of which, including breath control, simple meditation, and the adoption of specific bodily postures, is widely practiced for health and relaxation.

Yogi-One who practices yoga and has achieved a high level of spiritual insight. Let's visit the wise yogi, he may be able to offer us guidance by Spazizoner. Yogi is a dedicated practitioner of Yoga. Yoga, especially in the West, often refers to physical exercises (asanas) only. Here at The Yogin, we refer to Yoga as a holistic practice that includes but is not limited to Mantra, Asana, Pranayama and Meditation.

Yogin- a male person who is a Master of Yoga.

Yogini- a female master practitioner of tantra and yoga, as well as a formal term of respect for female Hindu or Buddhist spiritual teachers in the Indian subcontinent, Southeast Asia, and Greater Tibet.

Happiness- Happiness does not depend on what you have or who you are. It relies on what you think. Our thoughts have the most power over us. Our negative thoughts cause us to despair, sadness causes us to want things, and our positive thoughts demonstrate that we have everything we need. That is the key to happiness. Happiness is us; we just need to find it and embrace it.

Clarity - The ability to see things clearly only when you look in your heart, who looks outside dreams, who looks inside awakens.

Themes For classes

- Give yourself permission to let go while you are in a state of meditation. Avoid thinking about your day or worrying about tomorrow and stay grounded in the moment.
- Breath: pay attention to your breath. Pay attention to how your chest expands while inhaling gifts with love, gratitude, forgiveness, and compassion.
- When you exhale, let your breath go down to your stomach and feel how your stomach expands and fills up with oxygen.
- Feel how it nourishes your body.
- Observe how each breath cleanses the mind and the body.
- Stay present – set an intention for your practice. Intention is not about what we want, it's what is important to us.
- Practice self-affirmation

"I am beautiful

I am strong

I am truthful

I am enough

I am everything I want to be.

Each one of us is a miracle, and we need to know it."

Themes for classes

When we hold an awareness of what we need in the back of our minds, we direct our energy and the energy of the universe in that direction. When we make decisions, the universe conspires to make it happen.

Words can never hurt us unless we empower them.

The biggest problem is the disconnect from our center when we revert to self. All other things begin to fall away, and our lives begin to flow.

When we must remove clutter from our mind our greatest ability is to change our mind about ourselves.

The law of karma functions as a central motif in Hindu, Jaina, and Buddhism. It states that all actions have consequences. Those consquences will affect the doer of the action at some future time.

Cause and effect

We are always in mental chaos. We need to clear the mental clutter each day. We don't learn from experience. We learn what we choose to learn from experience.

Teaching moment: I learned I had to be willing to show up and shine.

Power yoga vinyasa- Power yoga, which is also known as Vinyasa yoga, is a fast-paced style of yoga that's focused on building strength and endurance. It is also an excellent form of yoga for burning calories, rinsing toxins, peeling away layers of tension and helping to clear away the heaviness we hold trapped in our body, poses, breaking down the painful but familiar holding pattern and returning our neutral body when patterns break new world energies.

The same stream of life that runs through my veins at night

Gratitude

- **Open Gratitude** – Often we are so busy chasing the things we don't have that we forget to notice the things we already have - the people in our lives and the fortunate circumstances in which we live.
- **Closed Gratitude** - is a powerful process for shifting your energy and bringing more of what you want into your life. Be grateful for what you already have, and you will be more attracted to good things.

Quotes Themes

Some people are sent to us for a quick lesson, some are sent to us for a seasonal lesson, and some are sent to us for lessons we are to be taught over a lifetime.

- **Energy:** Our physical body keeps us running.

Your body is a temple, and your soul is your inner sanctuary. Trust the self. It is your soul. Your body can't be neglected because it is the vessel that holds your soul. Your soul is also directly related to your emotions and mental and physical well-being, just as chemicals, pollution, electromagnetic waves and negative people deplete your energy body. Your energy is affected by exercise, diet and other lifestyle choices.

We are made from energy, and our soul is energy; the body is the carrier of energy in the physical world.

The Benefits of Ujjayi Breath

Ujjayi breath soothes the nervous system, calms the mind, and increases psychic sensitivity. It also relieves insomnia, slows down the heart rate, and lowers blood pressure. It is a tranquilizing pranayama, but it also has a heating effect, stimulating the process of oxidization at a cellular level.

Proper ujjayi breath allows us to stay longer and deeper in poses, helps us to sink deeper into meditation, and helps us to be grounded.

- Regulates heating of the body.

- Relieves headaches and sinus pressure.
- Strengthens the nervous and digestive systems.
- With each inhalation, notice how your chest expands, and with each exhalation let go of things and anxiety toward the unknown.
- Let go of what bothers you. Feel how the breath nourishes the body. Breathe deeply and purposefully and release anything that does not serve you.
- Breathe in life all the way to the bottom of your stomach. Inhale peace and exhale chaos.

Learning How to Breathe Properly

- Love meditation: "Being love" - being a loving human being is in our nature and is the basis of unconditional love.
- Progressively relax the body, and let all tension subside. Let thoughts come and go until they gradually fade away to reach a state of mindful tranquility. Focus on your breath as soon as you lose yourself. Avoid space and time references such as when you need to go, what happened yesterday, and what should be done tomorrow.
- Accept intuitive impressions. Absorb all your visions and new ideas without any mental reaction while maintaining alertness to prevent dizziness. By concentrating on your breath, you can explore the deeper meaning of your vision.
- Savasana. With closed eyes imagine a warm place in the sun. It is bright, and the sun radiates in all directions. Imagine yourself standing in the warm sand. Feel your feet touching the sand and the water and allow that image to bring tranquility and awareness.
- Breathing exercises can be completed sitting in the lotus pose, standing, or laying down on the mat.

Pranayama is a breath-control technique. In Sanskrit, pran means life, and ayama means way. Pranayama can help you regulate your system, alter your mood, and offer longevity. The main components of Pranayama are inhalation, exhalation and retention. Pranayama always begins with inhalations and exhalations. This strengthens the lungs and balances the nervous system, preparing the body to hold the breath [retention].

Practicing Pranayama regularly regulates energy flow to the 72 thousand nadis [channels through which consciousness flows] in our body, helping us improve our well-being.
- **Ujjayi breath**: Breathing evenly from both nostrils, also called the ocean breath.
- **Alternating nostrils**: alternating breath from one nostril to another.
- Setting an intention for your practice.

History of Yoga

What is Yoga?

- Yoga originated in India more than 5,000 years ago.
- Yoga means "yolk" or union:
    - Union of mind, body, spirit (vinyasa = body and breath)
    - Cessation of the mind – Osho
    - Physical and Spiritual Journey – the physical is seen as preparation for the spiritual; overall health benefits
    - Ashtanga Yoga - 8-limb path

8 Limbs of Yoga

- Yama
- Niyama
- Asana
- Pranayama
- Pratyahara
- Dharana
- Dhyana
- Samadhi

Yamas

- The Yamas deal with one's ethical standards and integrity
- The Yamas focus on behavior and how you carry yourself through life

Niyamas

- Sauca: purity, clearness of mind, speech, and body
- Santosa: contentment, acceptance of others and of one's circumstances as they are, optimism for self
- Tapas: perseverance, discipline, patience
- Svadhyaya: a study of self - self-reflection, involving the introspection of thoughts, speeches, and actions
- Isvarapranidhana: devotion, dedication to the ideal of pure awareness, true self.

Asana

- To be in good standing with oneself.
- Asanas, the postures practiced in yoga, comprise the third limb. In the yogic view, the body is a temple of spirit, the care of which is an important stage of our spiritual growth. Through the practice of asanas, we develop the habit of discipline and the ability to concentrate, both of which are necessary for meditation.
- There are all different kinds of Asanas!... Bikram, Hatha, Vinyasa, Kundalini, Restorative, Power, Gentle, Iyengar

Pranayama

- Prana=life force; breath
- Generally translated as breath control, this fourth stage consists of techniques designed to gain mastery over the respiratory process while recognizing the connection between the breath, the mind, and the emotions.
- As implied by the literal translation of pranayama, "life force extension," yogis believe that it not only rejuvenates the body but extends life itself. You can practice pranayama as an isolated technique (i.e., simply sitting and performing some breathing exercises) or integrate it into your daily hatha yoga routine.

Pratyahara

- Turning inward
- Pratyahara means withdrawal or sensory transcendence. It is during this stage that we make the conscious effort to draw our awareness away from the external world and outside stimuli. Keenly aware of, yet cultivating a detachment from our senses, we direct our attention internally. The practice of pratyahara provides us with an opportunity to step back and take a look at ourselves. This withdrawal allows us to objectively observe our cravings: habits that are perhaps detrimental to our health and which likely interfere with our inner growth.

Dharana

- Concentration...
Having relieved ourselves of outside distractions, we can now deal with the distractions of the mind itself. The practice of concentrating on a single mental object such as a specific energetic center in the body, an image, or the silent repetition of a sound. We, of course, have already begun to develop our powers of concentration in the previous three stages of posture, breath control, and withdrawal of the senses. In Asana and Pranayama, although we pay attention to our actions, our attention travels. In pratyahara, we become self-observant; now, in Dharana, we focus our attention on a single point. Extended periods of concentration naturally lead to meditation.

Dhyana

- Meditation or contemplation
- The uninterrupted flow of concentration
- Although concentration (dharana) and meditation (Dhyana) may appear to be one and the same, a fine distinction exists between these two stages. Where dharana practices one-pointed attention, Dhyana is ultimately a state of being keenly aware without focus. At this stage, the mind has been quieted and is in stillness. It produces few or no thoughts. It takes strength and stamina to reach this state of stillness, it's not easy. But don't give up. While this may seem like a difficult, if not impossible, task, remember that yoga is a process. Even though we may not attain the "picture perfect" pose or the ideal state of consciousness, we benefit at every stage of our progress.

Samadhi

- "A state of ecstasy" - Patanjali
- At this stage, the meditator merges with their point of focus and transcends the Self altogether. The meditator comes to realize a profound connection to the Divine, an interconnectedness with all living things. With this realization comes to the "peace that passes all understanding," the experience of bliss and being at one with the Universe.
- On the surface, this may seem to be a rather lofty, "holier than thou" kind of goal. However, if we pause to examine what we want to get out of life, wouldn't joy, fulfillment, and freedom somehow find their way onto our list of hopes, wishes, and desires? What Patanjali has described as the completion of the yogic path is what, deep down, all human beings aspire to: peace. We also might give some thought to the fact that this ultimate stage of yoga - enlightenment - can neither be bought nor possessed. It can only be experienced, the price of which is the continual devotion of the aspirant.

Stop and Discuss

- What is your personal experience or relationship to yoga practice?
- How can you connect the principles of the 8-limbed path to your everyday life?

Sanskrit

- One of the 14 original languages of India
- Postures named in Sanskrit; many have a story or a "legend" as well
- Why don't we use ONLY Sanskrit when teaching?

Benefits of Yoga

- BKS Iyengar: very sickly as a child, used yoga to regain his health. He was still practicing 3 hours of asana daily at the age of 90.
- Yoga affects the systems of the body to prevent and heal disease
- http://www.yogajournal.com/health/1634
- Energy release; balancing yin and yang; people come to yoga to balance energy levels (high energy to release, low energy to gain). How do you feel before and after yoga?

Stop and Discuss

- What is your personal definition of Yoga? What does Yoga mean to you?
- Start to think about your intention as a yoga teacher. Just as you set an intention before your yoga practice, it is important to have an intention as a teacher. What kind of energy and support do you hope to bring to your students?

PNF stretching

PNF is a stretching technique utilized to increase range of movement (ROM) and flexibility. PNF increases ROM by increasing the length of the muscle and increasing neuromuscular efficiency. PNF stretching has been found to increase ROM in trained as well as untrained, individuals.

There are three different types of PNF stretches

Contract-Relax Method

This involves contracting, holding, relaxing, and then stretching the targeted muscle group.

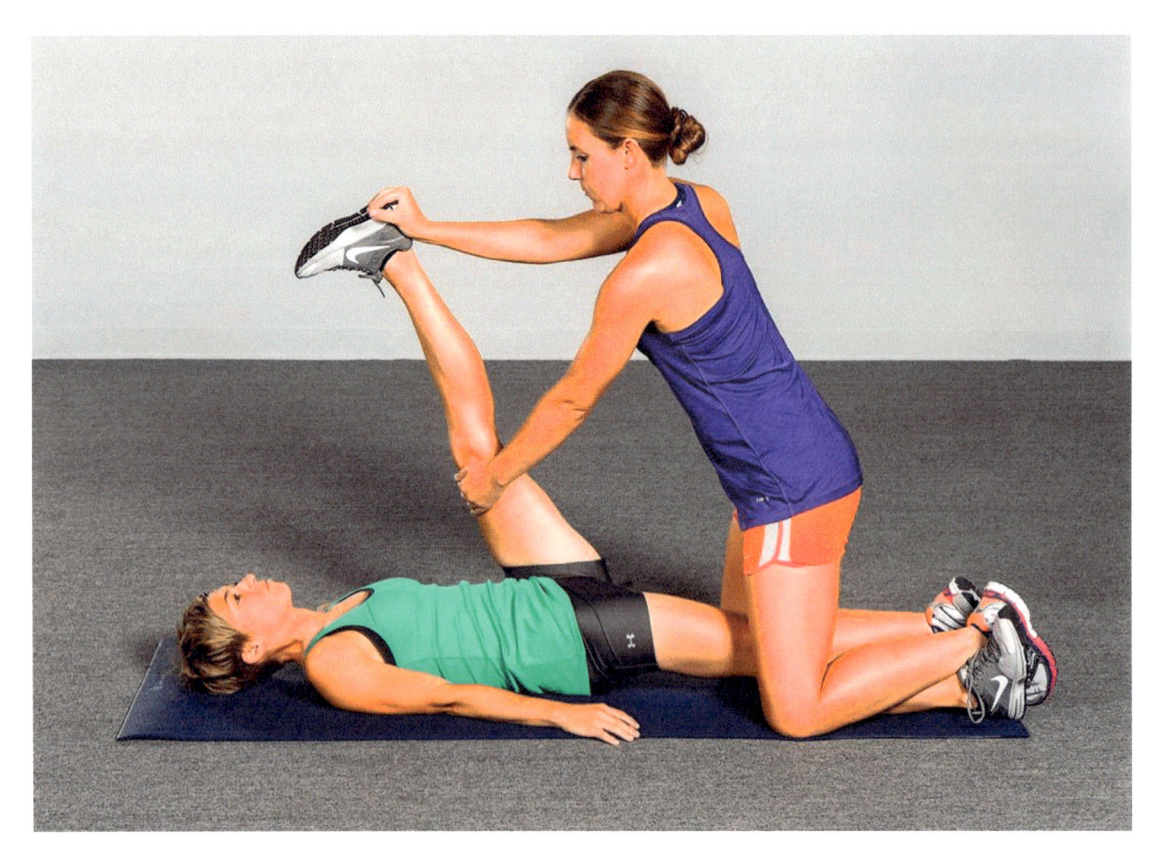

Antagonist-Contraction Method

Involves static or dynamic contraction of the opposite muscle group before stretching the targeted muscles and is followed by a static or dynamic stretch.

Static stretch

The holding of a muscle in an extended position for a period of time.

Dynamic stretch

An active movement that brings joints and muscles through their full range of motion.

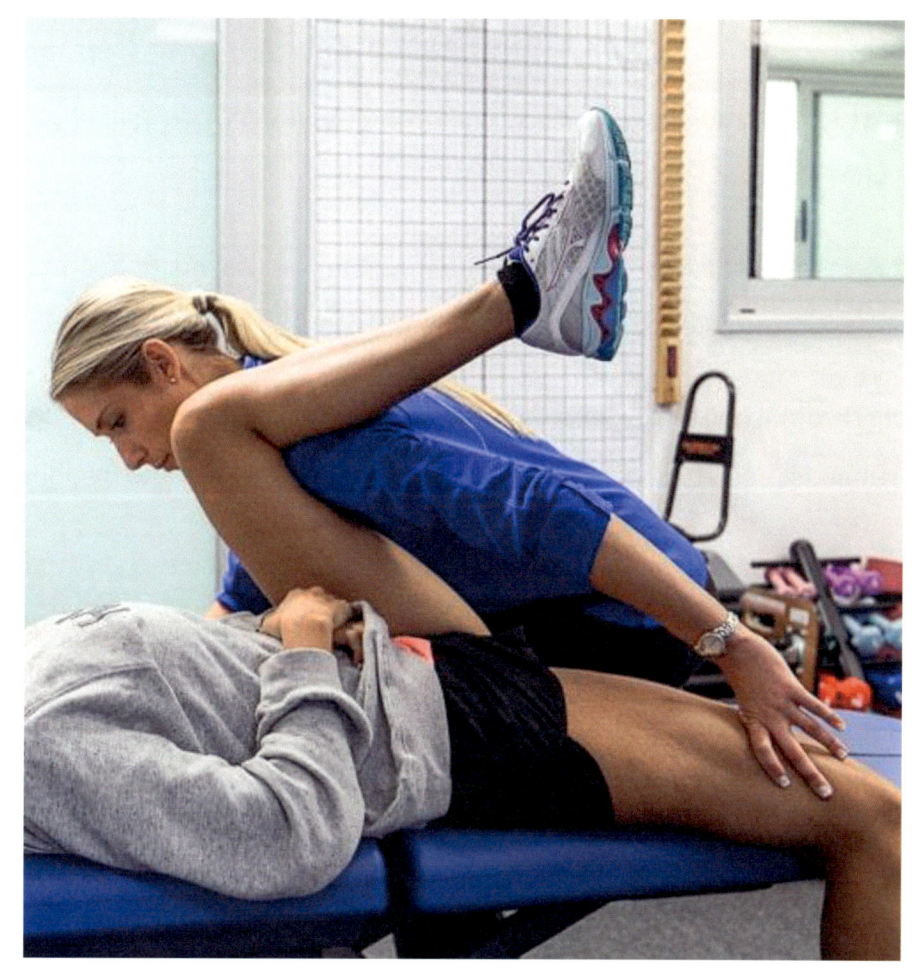

Contract-Relax-Antagonist-Contract Method

A combination of CR and AC. (Sometimes called **hold-relax-agonist-contraction**.)

Benefits of PNF Stretching

PNF stretching can improve your range of motion or ROM. It can also boost your muscle flexibility and strength.

By stretching or lengthening the muscle spindles and Golgi tendon organs (GTO) through PNF, you can increase your ROM.

Boosts ROM. Research indicates that PNF stretching may be the most effective method of stretching to increase your ROM.

Boost smuscle flexibility. Studies have shown that PNF can increase muscle flexibility. In particular, PNF can boost hamstring and lower leg (gastrocnemius) muscle flexibility.

Boosts muscle strength. PNF can boost the strength of your muscles. A study shows how vertical jumping and throwing distance can improve by more than double when athletes do PNF stretching twice a week for eight weeks.

Poses to get you grounded

In the Western world, spring is viewed as a time of hope, possibility, and rebirth. During spring, we might feel overwhelmed; one day, snow, the next sunny, and coasts off toasty. It forces us out of the cozy comfort zone we've developed over the winter.

But there is also an urge to refresh and rejuvenate that comes from deep inside. Finding your center is not always easy. It involves living in the present and gaining awareness of time and pressure. It means learning to embrace the uncertainty of life.

Healing begins with grounding poses.

Tadasana

Mountain pose is also called tree pose.

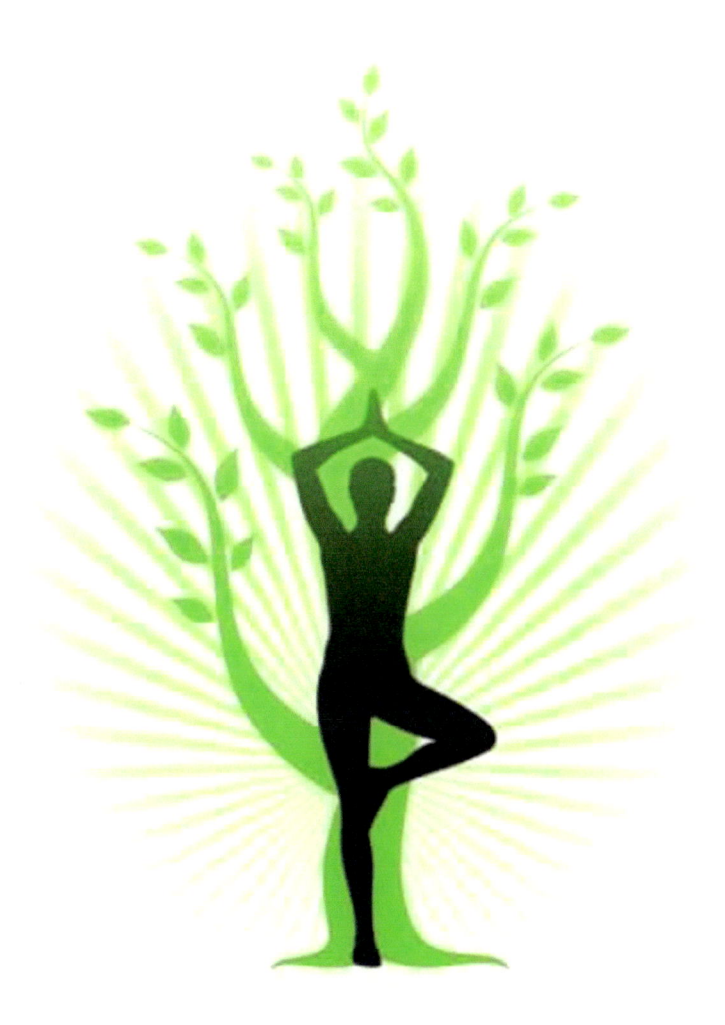

In this pose, firmly rooted to the ground while the crown of your head acknowledges the sky. While in tadasana, imagine your feet sprouting roots that grow deeply into the ground.

Imagine a great ancient tree with a wide trunk, whose roots dig deep into the earth and spread wide, holding the tree in place and physically connecting it to the earth. From the earth, the trees receive everything they need to sustain themselves. The tree is secure in this knowledge and, day after day, reaches its branches toward the sky to happily drink in the sunshine. Now imagine yourself as that tree with a deep woody root base that connects you to the physical world; just as a tree drinks in the sunshine, you drink in the nourishing air around you. Each breath gives you a taste of sunshine that gives you a sense of well-being. This is the essence of balancing the chakra system.

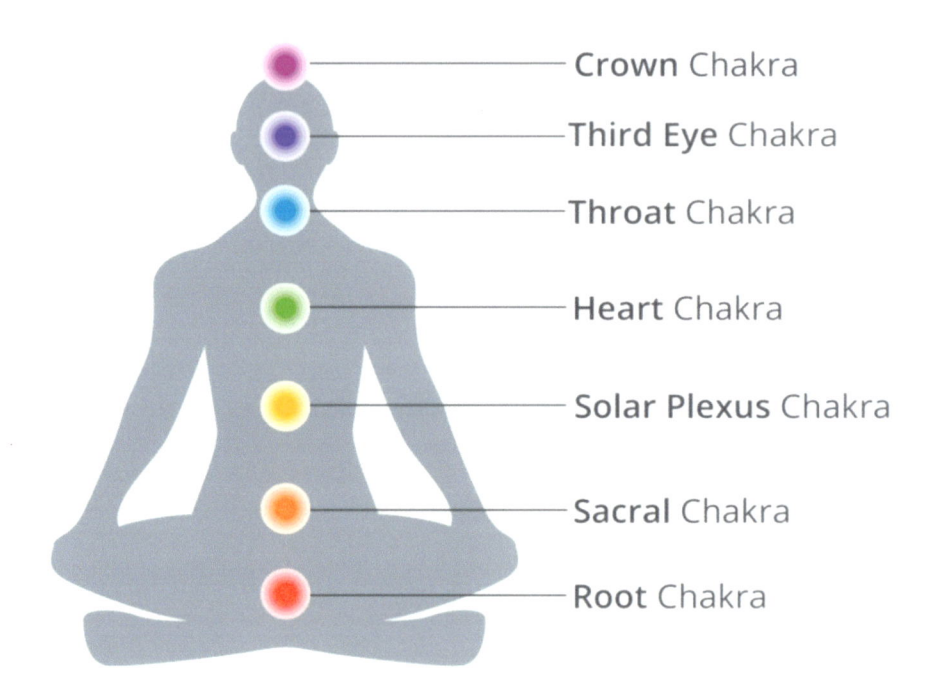

Now imagine that the tree is in a hurricane and the roots slowly become drenched with excessive water from the storm. They begin to pull out of the mud while some of the tree branches break and fall to the ground. The wind whips at the leaves, carrying some of them into the air. The tree remains after the storm but also no longer stable on the earth. There is a sense of imbalance.

The chakra system holds your body's energy (or prana-life force), and your actions can help keep it in balance. The Sanskrit word chakra translates to a wheel or disk. In yoga, meditation, and Ayurveda, this term refers to wheels of energy throughout the body.

The chakra are subtle energy centers, like wheels within the body. The chakras spin at the speed of light, enhancing the colors combined to form the auras that surround each of us. They connect with each other and with the cosmos.

There are seven to eight major chakras in the body. Their location corresponds to regions of the body where nerves collect and electrical activity is high, such as brachial and sacral plexus - primary chakra, and the elbows and the knees which are minor chakras.

The flow of energy in the chakras can become blocked by life events through the activity of the autonomic nervous system. For example, when we habitually assume defensive postures in response to harmful stimulation, we block the flow of energy in the chakra. Hatha yoga reverses this process, and this stimulates the chakras, allowing them to spin freely.

Kundalini awakening refers to the unblocking of the flow of energy through and between the chakras, this process can accrue instantly from contact with a master who awakens the student's awareness of his or her potential. Classically this occurs through touch but can occur with a glance and even through the presence of the master. This is known as shaktipat, the transmission of the psycho-spiritual energy as human consciousness that transforms with age. More and more people spontaneously experience varying degrees of kundalini awakening.

Kundalini awakening is akin to tapping into a high-voltage line that requires careful preparation. Hatha yoga prepares the practitioner and awakens the kundalini at the same time.

Asanas connect the body and mind. Breathing techniques connect consciousness and unconsciousness. Chakra meditation connects individuals to the vibrational energy of the cosmos. Spend a few moments gazing at this image of the chakra, and then take time to meditate as you visualize the chakras. They will appear as a subtle but scintillating light within you.

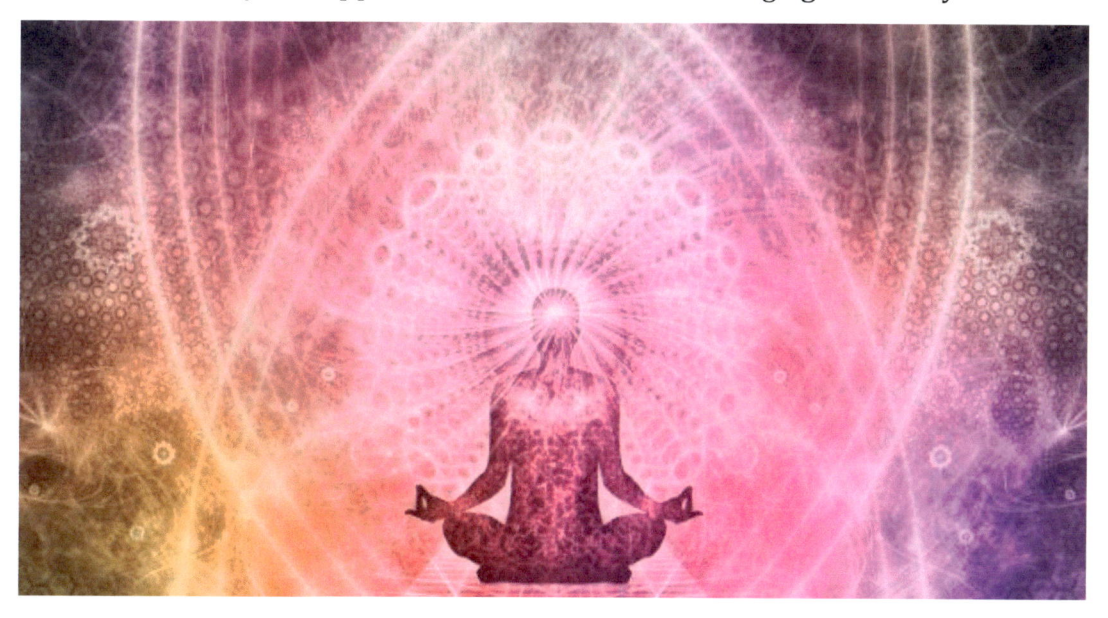

Here is an excellent exercise for you since you can find out what each chakra means online. Please describe each chakra, its effects, color, and what Yoga poses may balance it out.

You can also google essential oils for each Chakra and write about them.

Please Email it to Vyoga4u@gmail.com.

Second Exercise

I will give you a list of poses (asanas) in Sanskrit

Please attach a

 picture for the pose and explanation.

Utkatasana

Virabadrasana

VIrakasana

Utkatasana

VIrabodrasana 1, 2, 3

Sirsasana right and left

Konasanakatichakrasana

Dandasana

Uttanasana

Makarasana Locust pose

Sahaja Mayurasana

Gomukhasana

Makarasana

Also, behind every pose, there is a history of mysticism. Please write about at least 2 poses and their mystical story.

You can find all the information on Google.

Please send responses to Vyoga4u@gmail.com.

Third Exercise

Please write about how you found Yoga.

Have you ever practiced aromatherapy during Yoga? If yes, please explain briefly.

Please send to Vyoga4u@gmail.com.

Essential oils and yoga: You can always incorporate essential oils during class or at the end of class. Your theme can also start with the use and introduction of essential oils.

Here are some ways to incorporate essential oils into your yoga class

- Pass oils around at the beginning of class and have students rub them on their feet, temples, or the backs of their necks.
- Spritz an essential oil blend throughout the space at the beginning and end of class.
- Diffuse oils in the space throughout the class.
- Give the students a spritz or application of the essential oil before or immediately after shavasana.

All ABOUT ANATOMY

Patanjali, the patron saint of yoga, said that mastery combines a balance of science and art. Knowledge of science is like the colors on an artist's palette - the greater the knowledge, the more colors are available. The body is the canvas, and the asanas are the art we create.

Introduction: it is not necessary to memorize hundreds of muscles and bones to experience the benefits of applying science to yoga. What is essential is the functional understanding of a manageable number of the key anatomic structures in their settings as they relate to hatha yoga.

The skeletal system is made up of bones and joints

Bones

Bones are not solid; they are filled with marrow and wrapped with an outer lining that can be bruised.

Periosteum is the skin of the bone, comprised of ⅔. rigid tissues, ⅓ elastic tissues

Somewhat elastic, they move, bow, and slightly bend. Inflexible structures are not sound shock absorbers.

Bones grow and strengthen with resistance and gravitational pressure.

Standing strengthens bones more than lying down.

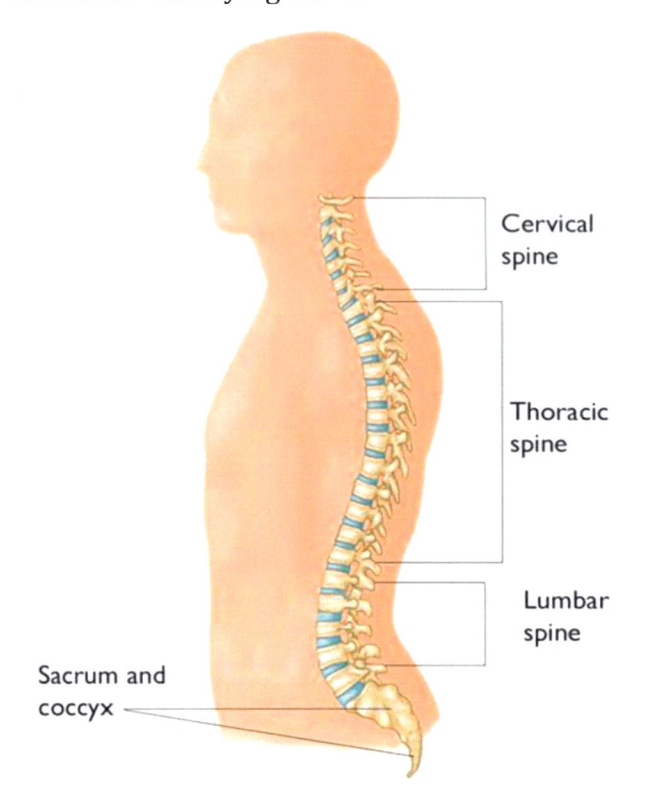

The human skeletal system

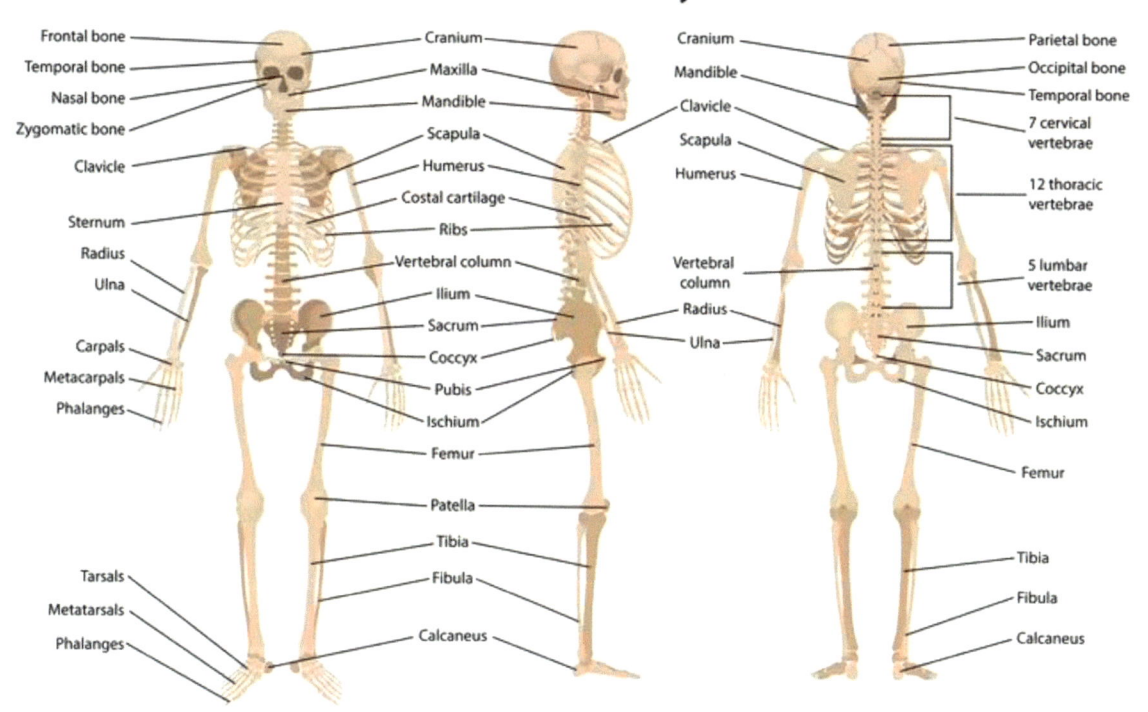

Joints

Joints are where bone meets bone. A lot of friction and impact occurs here.

Compression

Ligaments connect bone to bone, and function to straighten and stabilize the joints passively.

Tendons connect muscles to bone.

As with bones, the shape of the joints reflects their function, and their function reflects their shape.

Joints come in a spectrum of shapes, depending on the mobility or stability they require

For example, the hip joint is a ball and socket, while the knee joint is a hinge.

A ball and socket hip joint confers the most incredible mobility in all planes. It is helpful for activities such as changing direction while walking or running (or reaching in various directions to grab something, as with the shoulder).

A hinge-type knee joint provides excellent stability and helps propel the body forward (or draw an object towards the body, as with the elbow).

Other joints, such as the intervertebral between the vertebrae, allow for limited mobility between individual vertebrae but more excellent stability to protect the spinal cord.

Mobility of the spinal column comes from the limited movement of...

(a) Pivot joint (between C1 and C2 vertebrae)

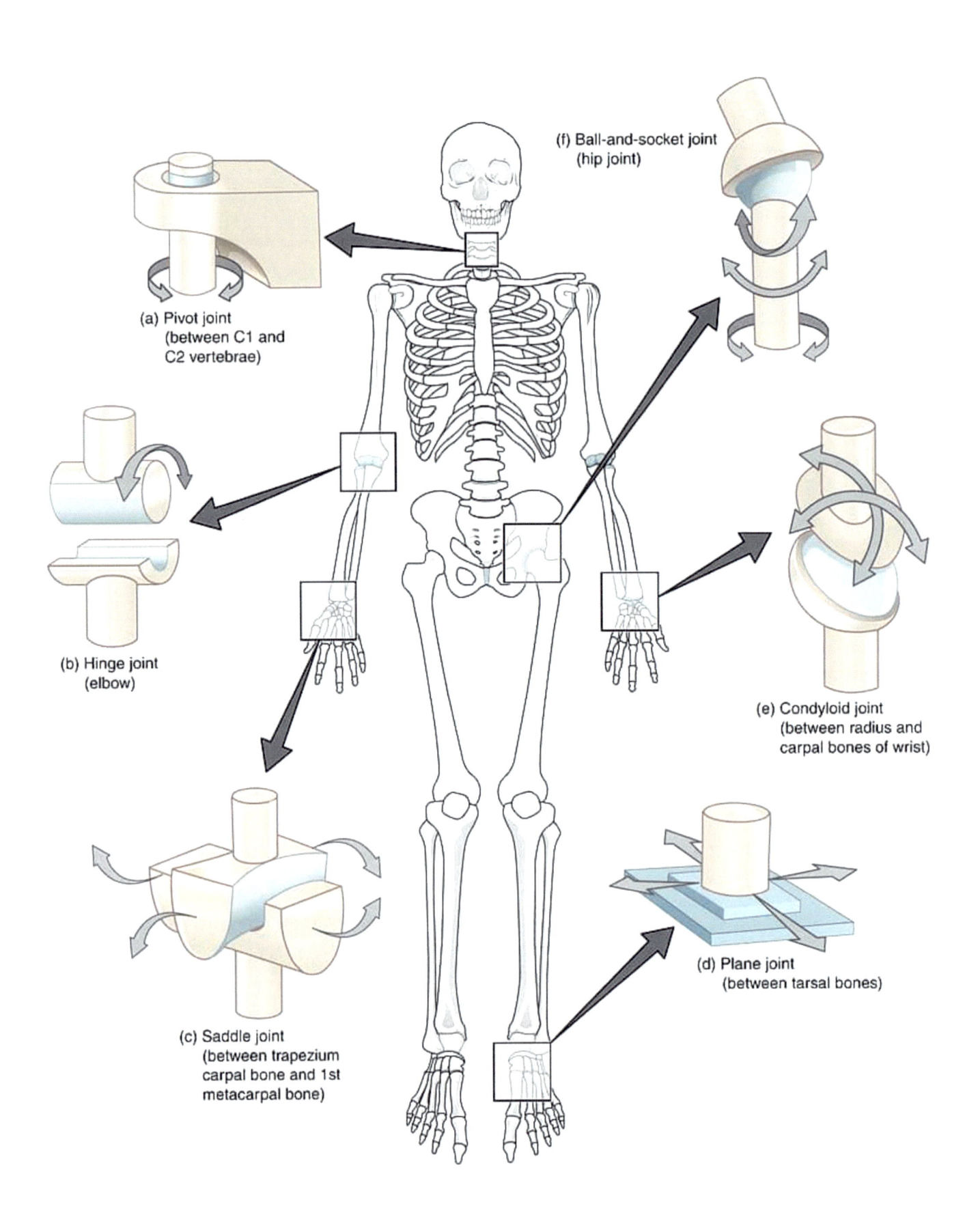

(b) Hinge joint (elbow)

(c) Saddle joint (between trapezium carpal bone and 1st metacarpal bone)

(d) Plane joint (between tarsal bones)

(e) Condyloid joint (between radius and carpal bones of wrist)

(f) Ball-and-socket joint (hip joint)

The articulating surfaces of the bones are covered by articular cartilage, a thin layer of hyaline cartilage. The walls of the joint cavity are formed by the connective tissue of the articular capsule. The synovial membrane lines the interior surface of the joint cavity and secretes the synovial fluid.

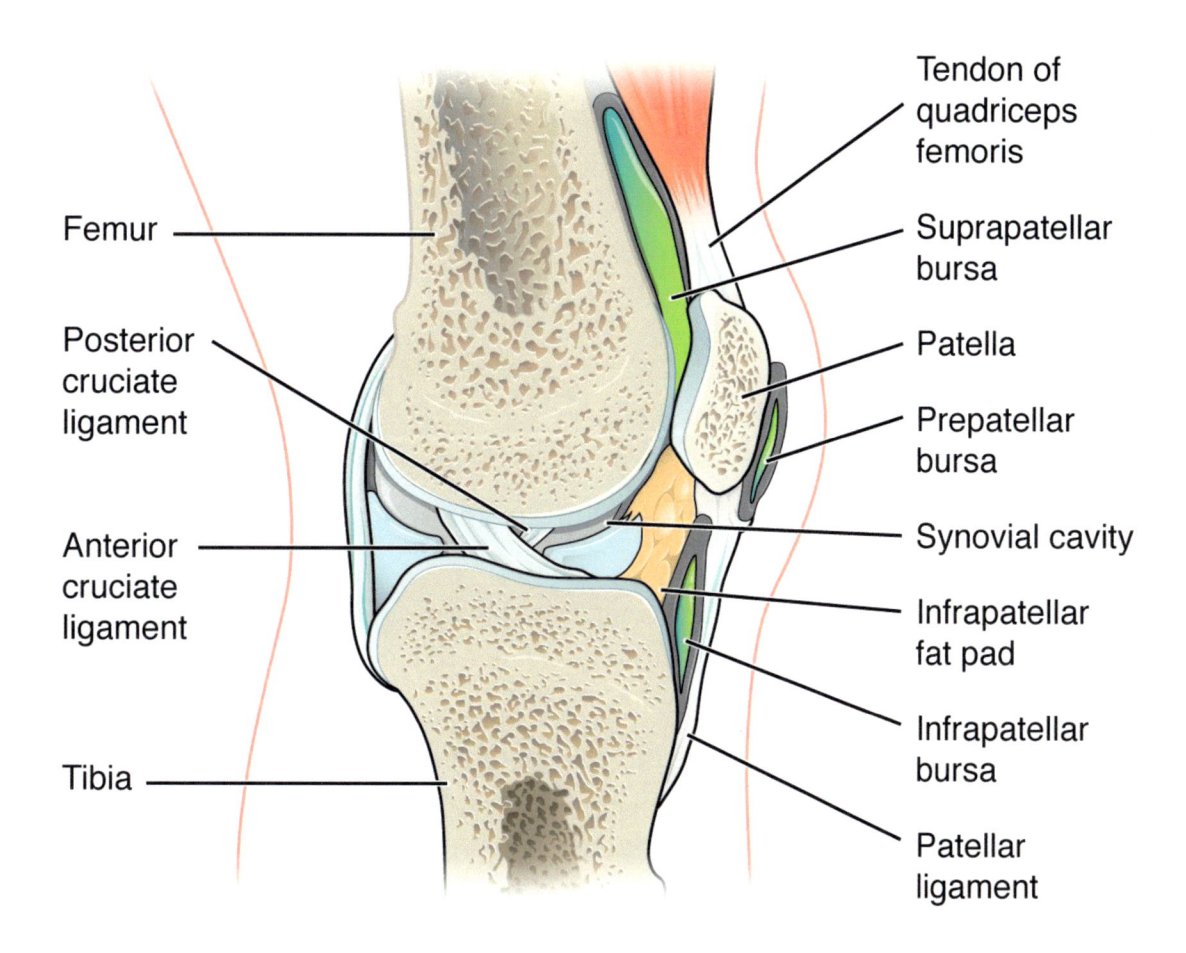

Joint Reaction Forces

The joint reaction forces and moments are distributed among the muscles that cross each joint. The muscles around the proximal joint are typically modeled as vectors acting along straight lines between the point of origin and the point of insertion.

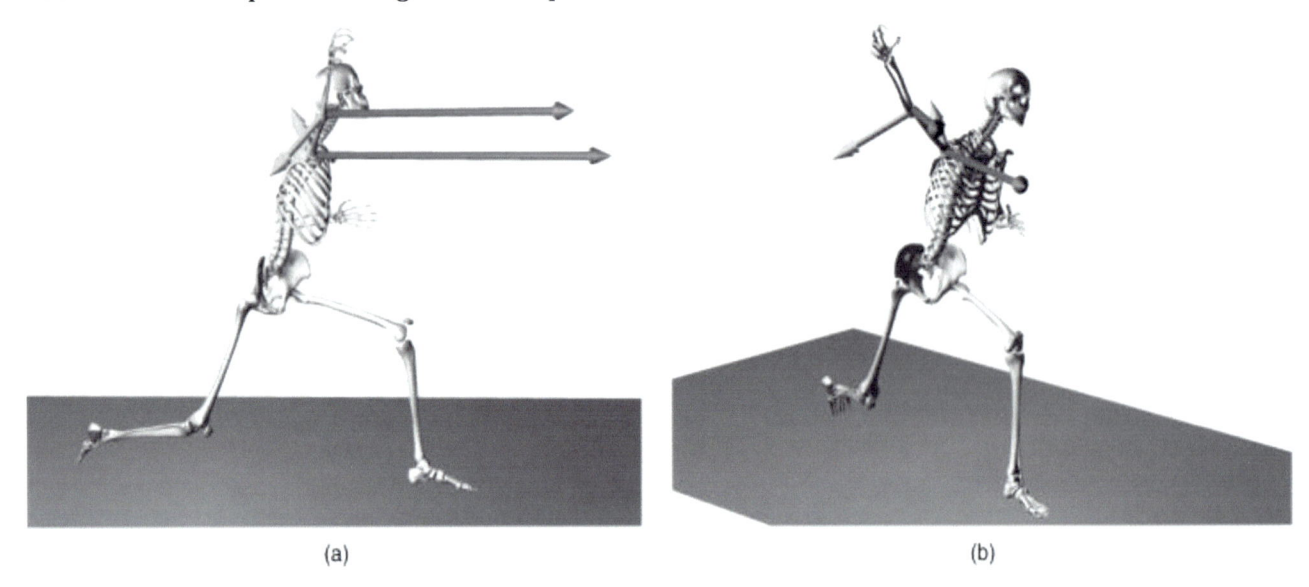

(a)   (b)

Joint reaction force is defined as the force generated within a joint in response to forces acting on the joint. In the hip, it is the result of the need to balance the moment arms of the body weight and abductor tension.

Joint reaction forces are opposing forces across the joint surface. To prevent injury, it's important to spread these forces over as much joint surface area as possible. Congruency of a joint is how well the surfaces fit and move with each other.

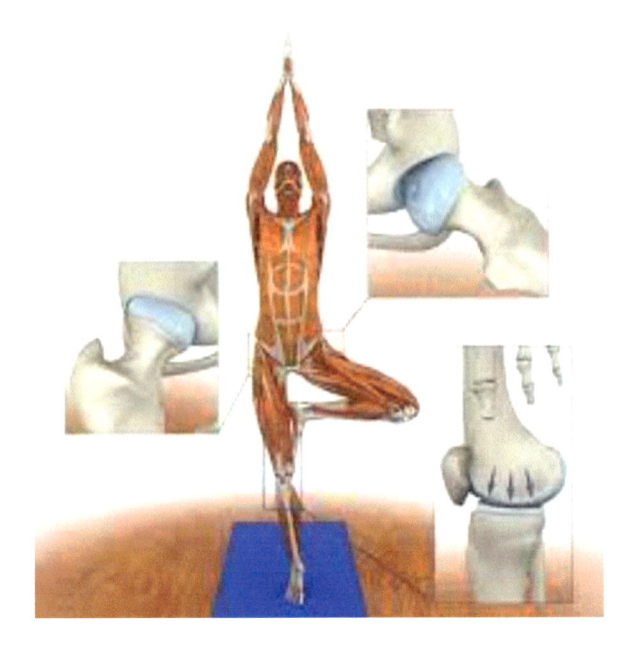

Muscular System

Muscles move by pulling bones. They are composed of thousands of muscle fibers, but not all of the fibers run in the same direction.

Depending on the orientation and attachment of the fibers, a muscle can pull in many directions.

Types of Muscle Action

- Concentric: shortening contraction. Example: The action of straightening your front leg (quad muscles) when coming out of Warrior 1.
- Eccentric: lengthening contraction (the negative in weightlifting). Example: The action of lowering your front leg (quad muscles) in Warrior 1
- Isometric: constant length and tension with movement, like pushing against a wall. Example: The action of holding Warrior 1 for five breaths.

Muscle Terminology

Agonist is equal to Prime Mover: This is the muscle performing the desired motion of the joint.

Antagonist: Muscles that perform the opposite motion of the desired motion (Example- biceps and triceps; quad and hamstring)

Synergist: Other muscles that participate in the desired motion.

To know which muscles must properly contract in a pose, we must also know which muscles are inhibiting the movement. If the antagonist does not relax, muscular contraction cannot occur (triceps holding/biceps struggle to lengthen). If the antagonist is contracting, then you create an isometric contraction or an inefficient contraction.

Fascia/Connective Tissue

Fascia is the "plastic wrap" of the body

- Wraps and connects everywhere
- Creates a web that supports, positions, and shapes the body
- Creates an integrated unit

Fascia surrounds all muscle fibers. It allows muscles to have more cross-sectional area and work in many directions and along many lines of pull.

Stagnant Fascia: With habitual inefficient posture, fascia can get thick and stuck, holding the body in misalignment.

- Muscle groups can get stuck together and work as an imbalance unit during some motions instead of allowing muscles to work separately.

Stretching muscles

Hence, when you stretch, the muscle fiber is pulled out to its full length by the sarcomere, and then the connective tissue takes up the remaining slack. When this occurs, it helps to realign any disorganized fibers in the direction of the tension.

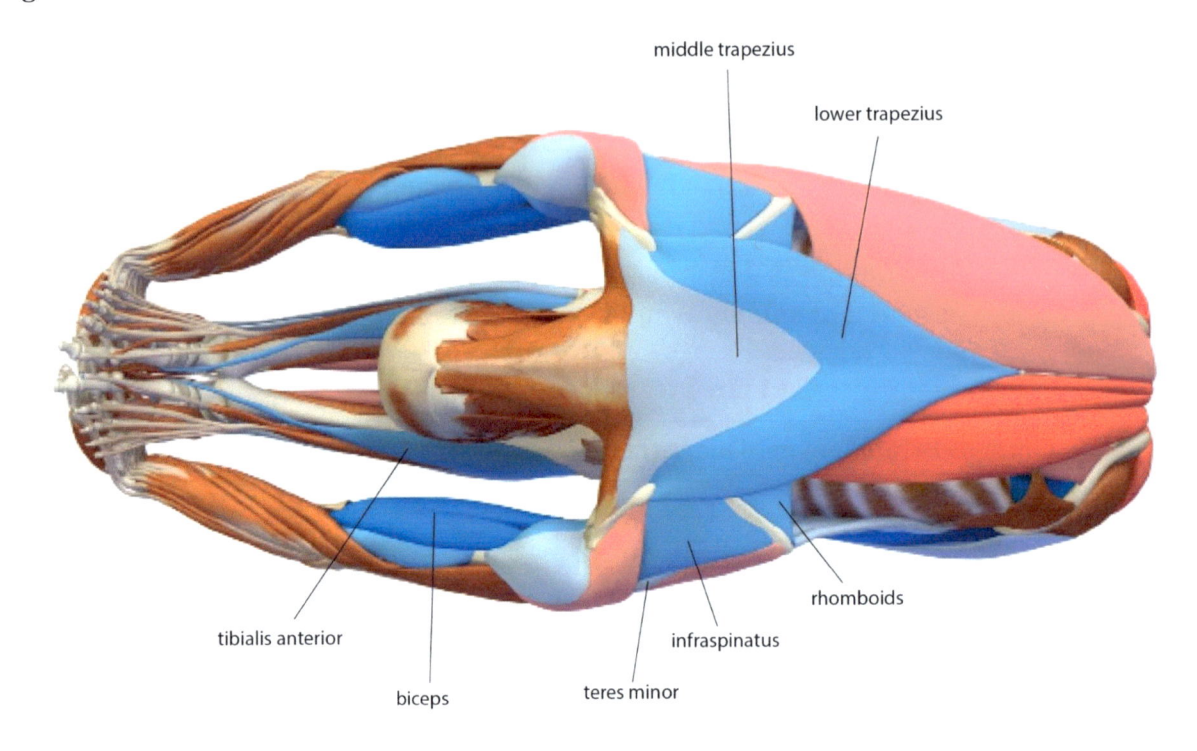

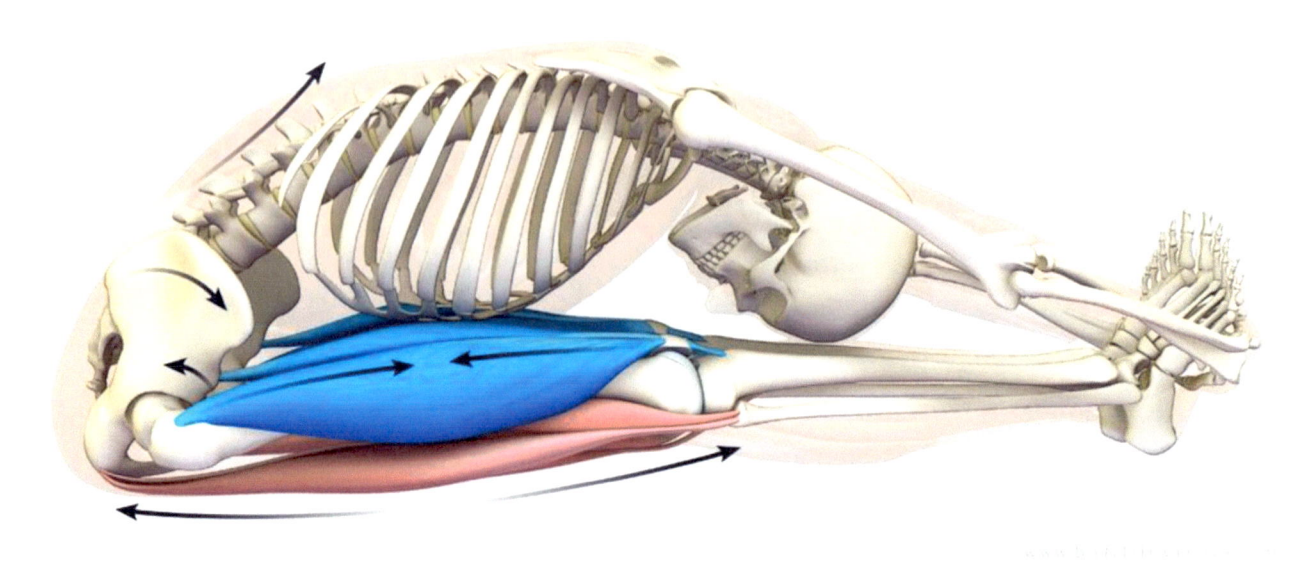

58

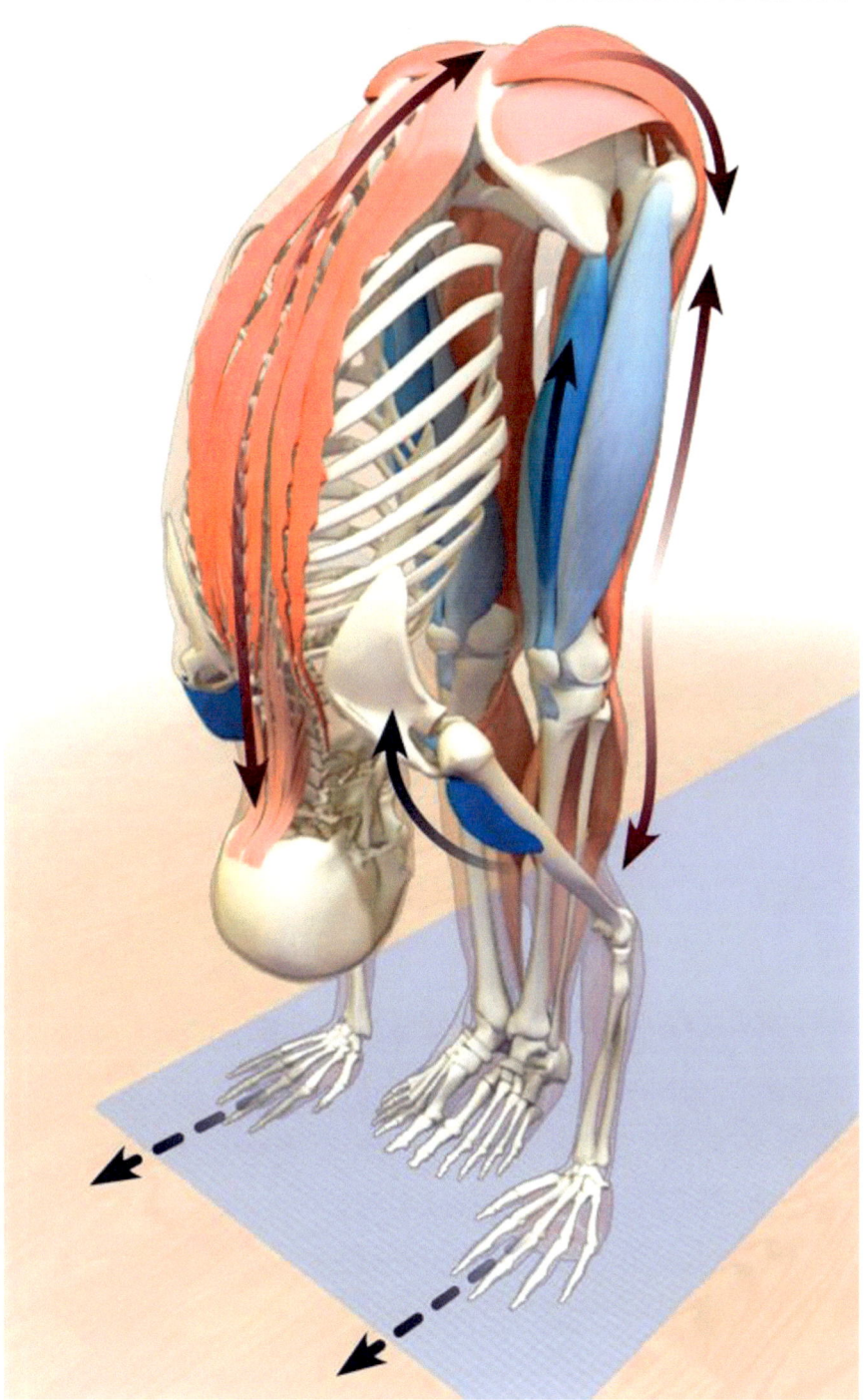

Facilitated stretching

Proprioceptive Neuromuscular Facilitation (PNF) is a stretching technique utilized to improve muscle elasticity and has been shown to have a positive effect on active and passive range of motion.

For example, if you wish to stretch the hamstrings, have the stretcher lie on her back on a mat or a treatment table and contract her quadriceps and psoas (hip flexors) to actively lift the leg as high as possible, keeping the knee straight. This stretches the hamstrings to their end range.

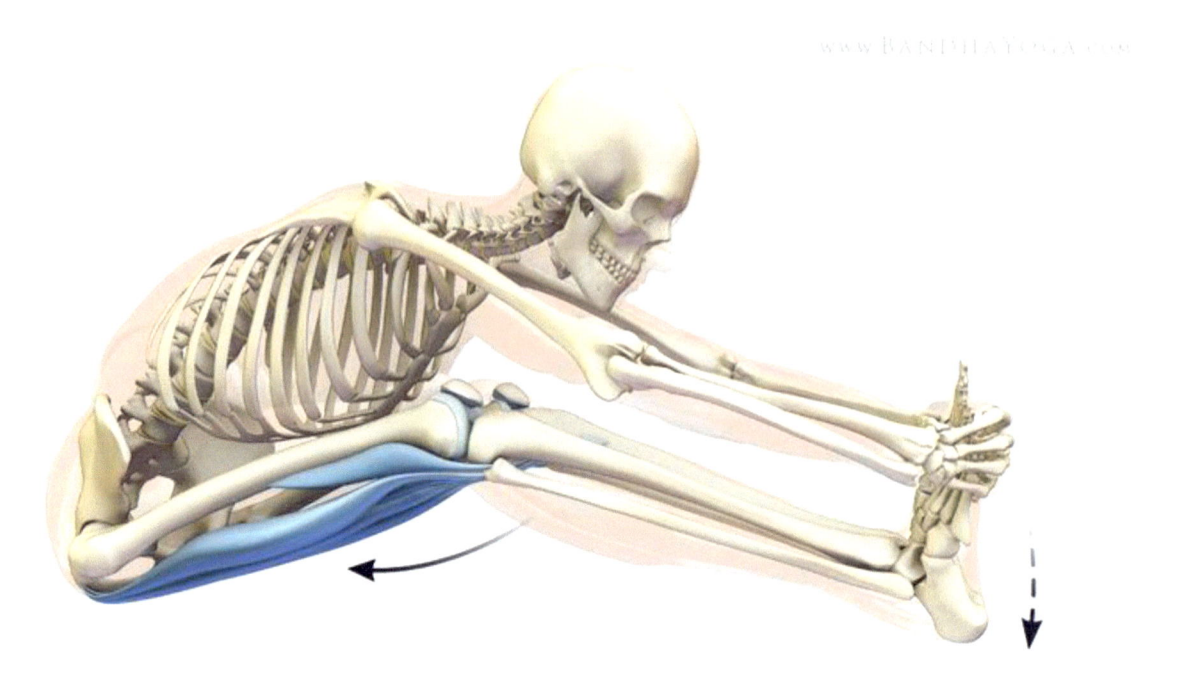

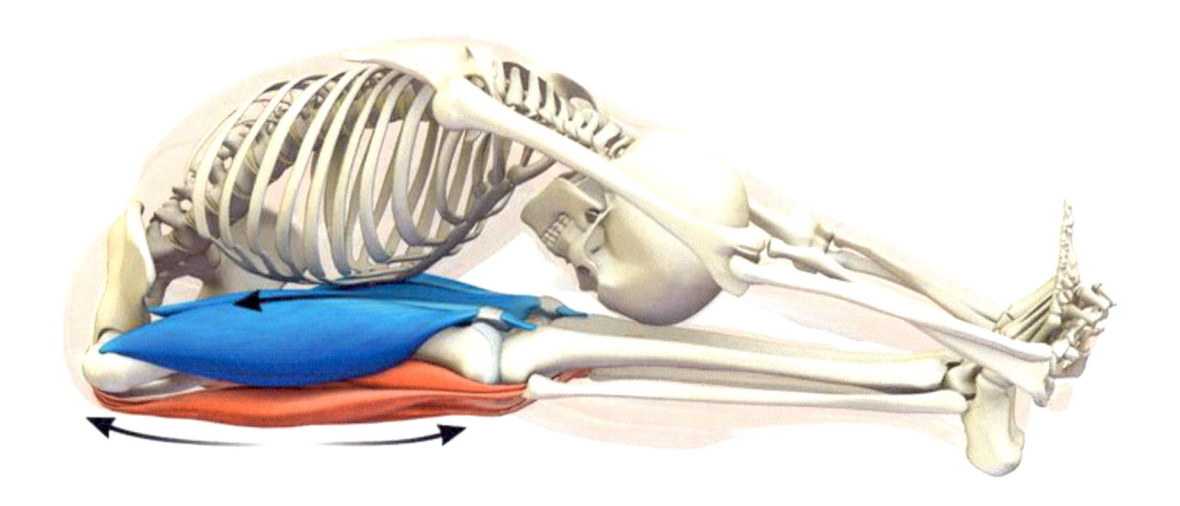

Dynamic Stretching

Dynamic stretches are a series of gentle arm and leg swings performed in a smooth, controlled manner. They involve continuous movement throughout the exercise and are considered more effective in "warming" up a muscle and promoting more blood flow to the region than static stretches.

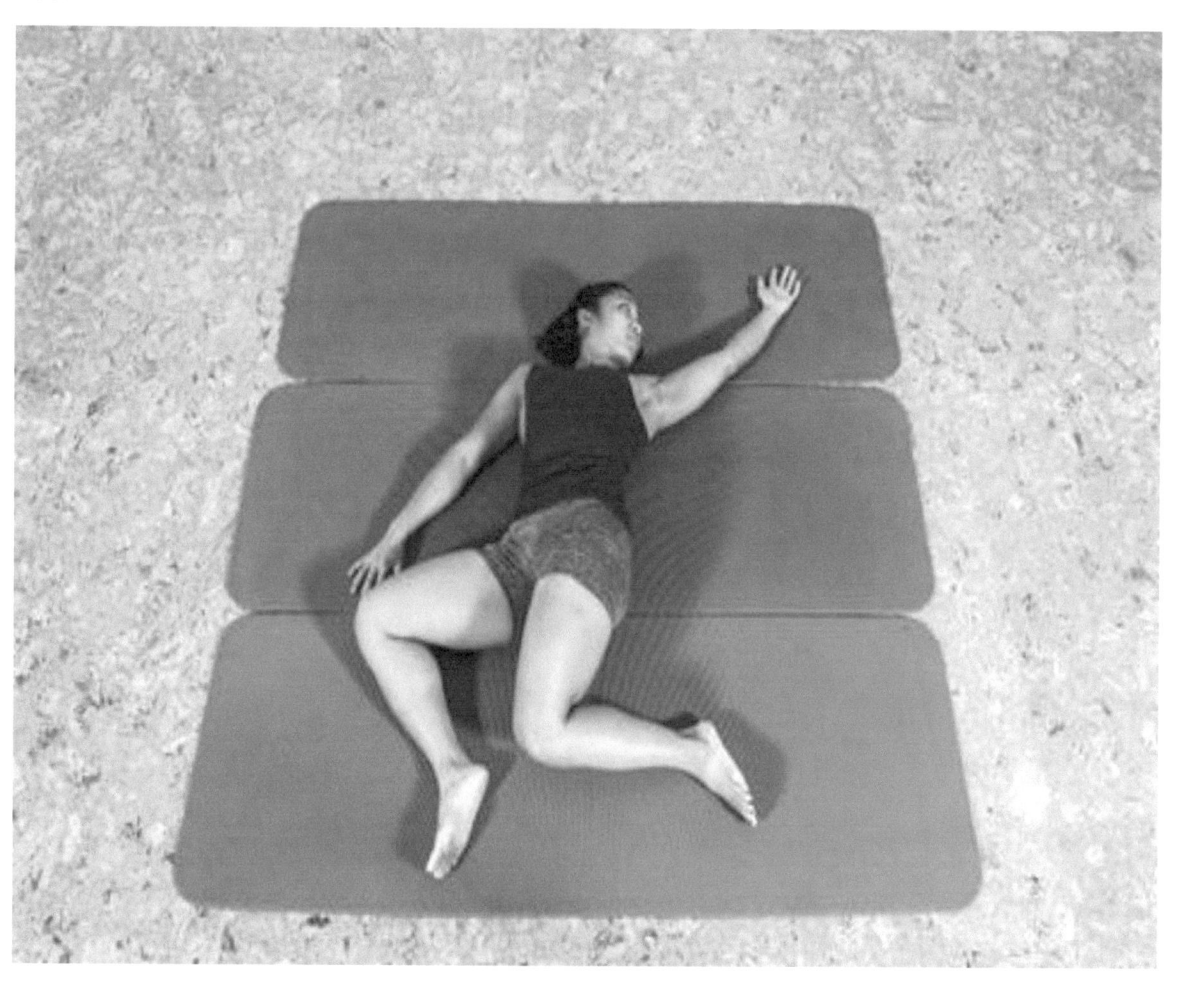

Pelvic Girdle and Thighs:

There are six external rotators of the hip

- Piriformis,
- Gemellus superior,
- Obturator internus,
- Gemellus
- Inferior
- Obturator externus
- Quadratus femoris

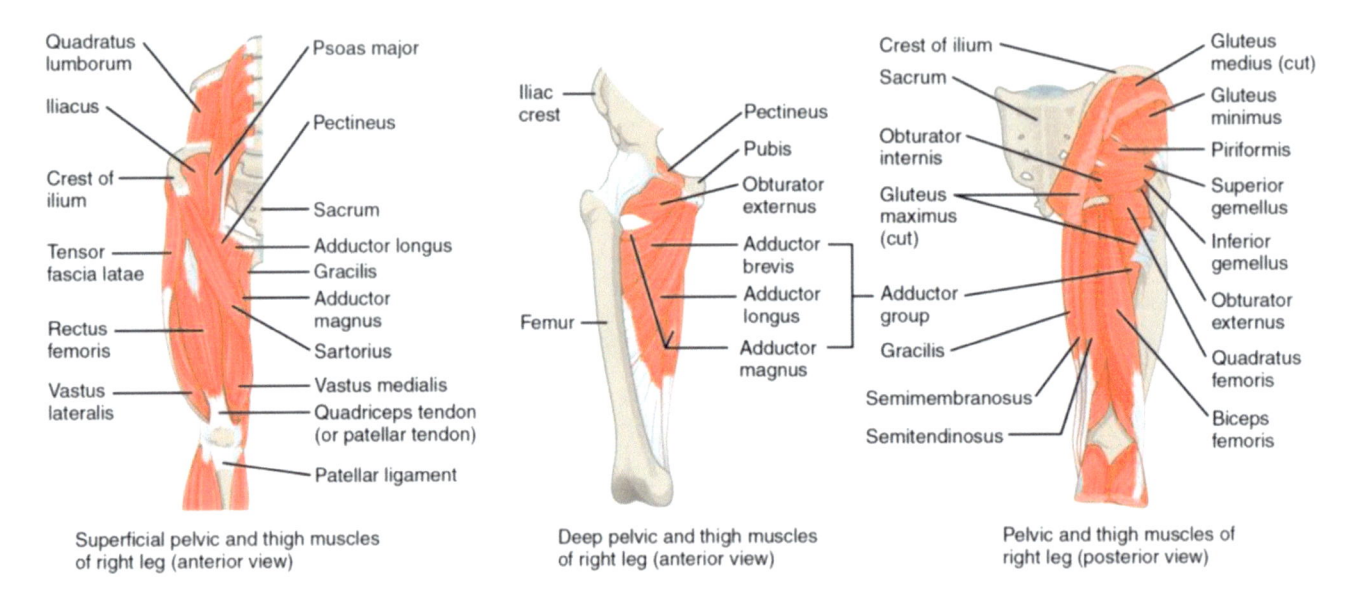

Iliopsoas:

The iliopsoas muscle is the primary flexor of your hip joint. It's made up of three muscles: the iliacus, the psoas major, and the psoas minor. These muscles work together to flex your hips, as well as stabilize your hips and lower back during activities like walking, running, and rising from a chair.

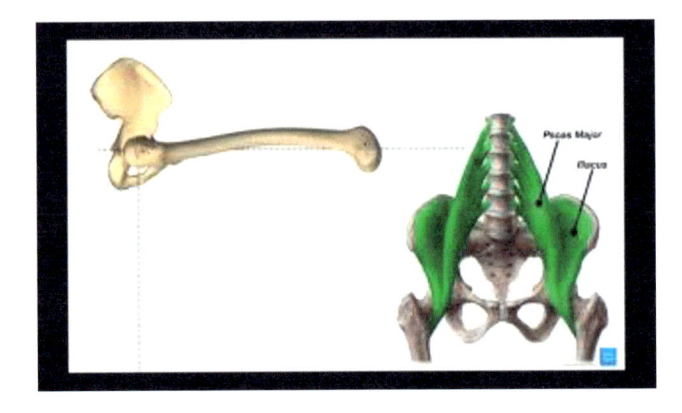

The iliopsoas muscle is the primary hip flexor. It assists in the external rotation of the hip joint, playing an essential role in maintaining the strength and integrity of the hip joint. It is vital for correct standing or sitting lumbar posture, and plays a critical role during walking and running.

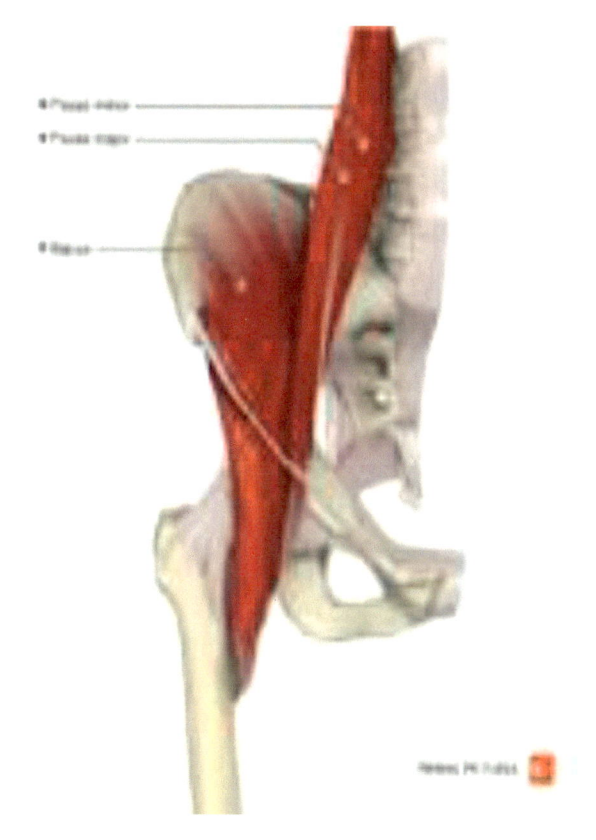

The iliopsoas works in relationship with its synergists (muscles doing the same action) and antagonists (muscles doing the opposite action) to allow a healthy range of flexion, extension, adduction, abduction, and rotation of the hip joint, as well as the anterior and posterior tilt of the pelvis.

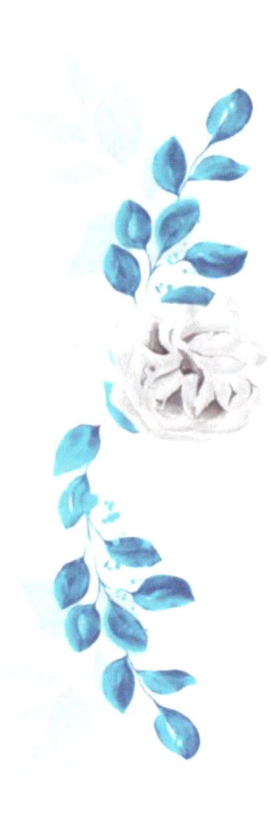

THE MIGHTY PSOAS – THE MUSCLE OF THE SOUL

Psoas is short for iliopsoas.
The iliopsoas is called many things:
  The Trap, a Storage Unit, and even the Garbage Dump.

Fight-Flight-Freeze Muscle
The antidote to Fight-Flight-Freeze is our **Relaxation Response**

A healthy iliopsoas is important for all the movements that you make in daily life. It is the only muscle that connects our upper and lower half therefore, it **involves absolutely everything we do**.

It's vital to strengthen, stretch, and lengthen these muscles to awaken and release the area as well as **prevent future injuries and soul wounds.**

YogaFaith.org

The Psoas Awakening Series synergistically combines the standing poses to awaken the psoas muscle. We do this by first contracting the psoas in poses that face forward, and then in poses that face the side. We complete the series with twisting postures.

Remembering that this muscle is usually "hidden" in the unconscious part of the brain, we must first isolate the psoas in each pose, bringing it back to consciousness.

I use the technique of isometric contraction to isolate and awaken a dormant muscle. This technique requires an understanding of the action of the various muscles. For example, the psoas acts to flex the hip, i.e., contracting the psoas either bends the trunk forward or draws the knee up. If you are contracting your psoas on one side, it laterally flexes your trunk. It also synergizes the external rotation of the hip.

Isolate your psoas (and its synergist muscles) by attempting to flex the trunk or by trying to lift the leg. Accentuate this by resisting the action. Check out Figure 1 below for how to do this with Trikonasana. You can then transport the technique to other poses.

Figure 1: Engaging your psoas.

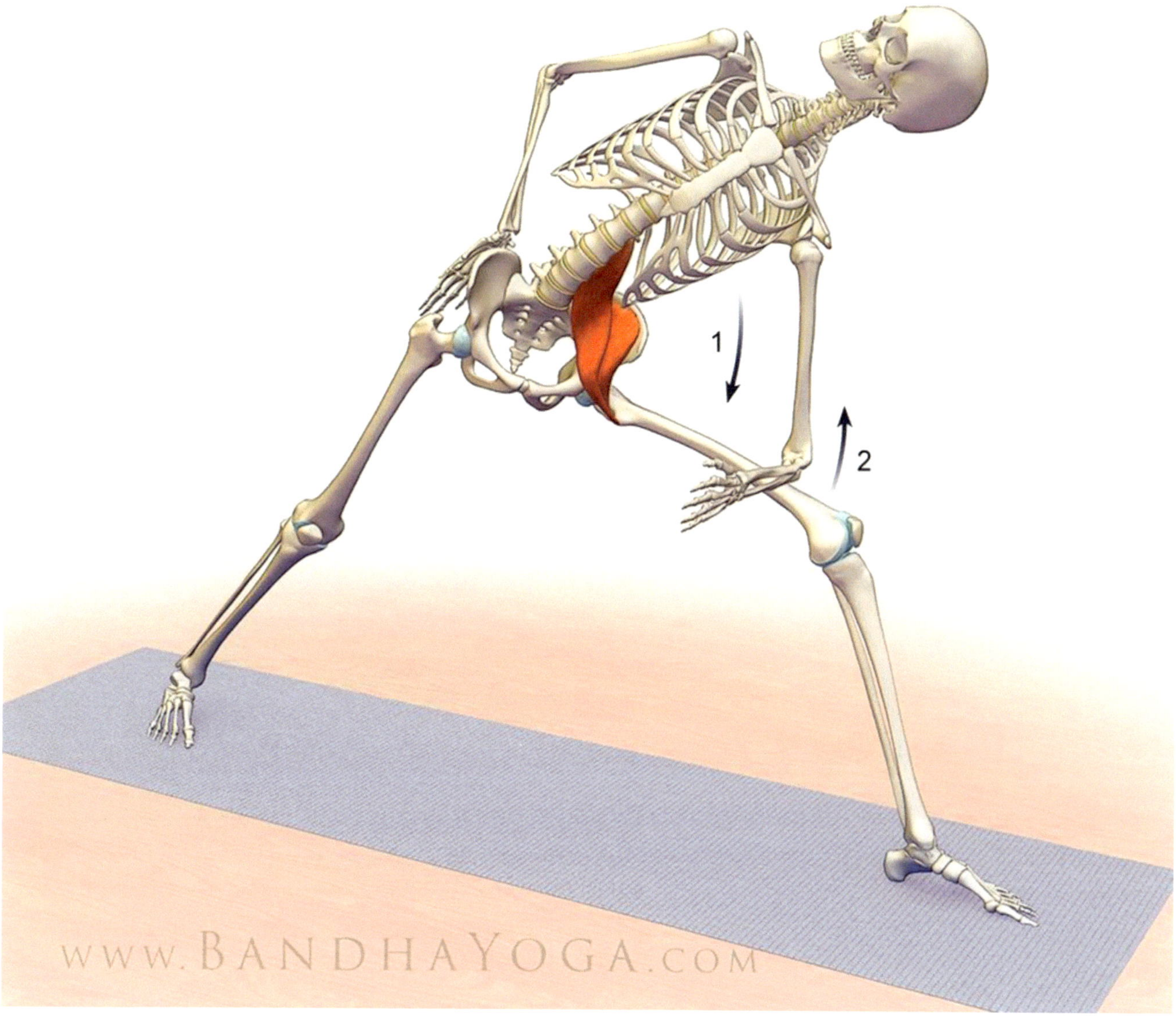

Place your elbow on your thigh as shown. Then, attempt to press the elbow down against your thigh by flexing your trunk to the side (Arrow 1). Relax for a moment and then attempt to lift your leg straight up against your elbow. Finally, press down with your trunk and try to lift your leg against your elbow simultaneously. Neither your trunk nor your thigh will move in either of these actions, but you will feel your psoas muscle engage in your pelvis.

Remember, it is not necessary to use maximum contraction. Work with around twenty percent of your max force. Use gradual engagement with these cues and ease into the contraction. Similarly, ease out of the movement and pose.

This general sequence will be repeated for each pose throughout the series.

Figure 2: Co-contracting your glutes and psoas.

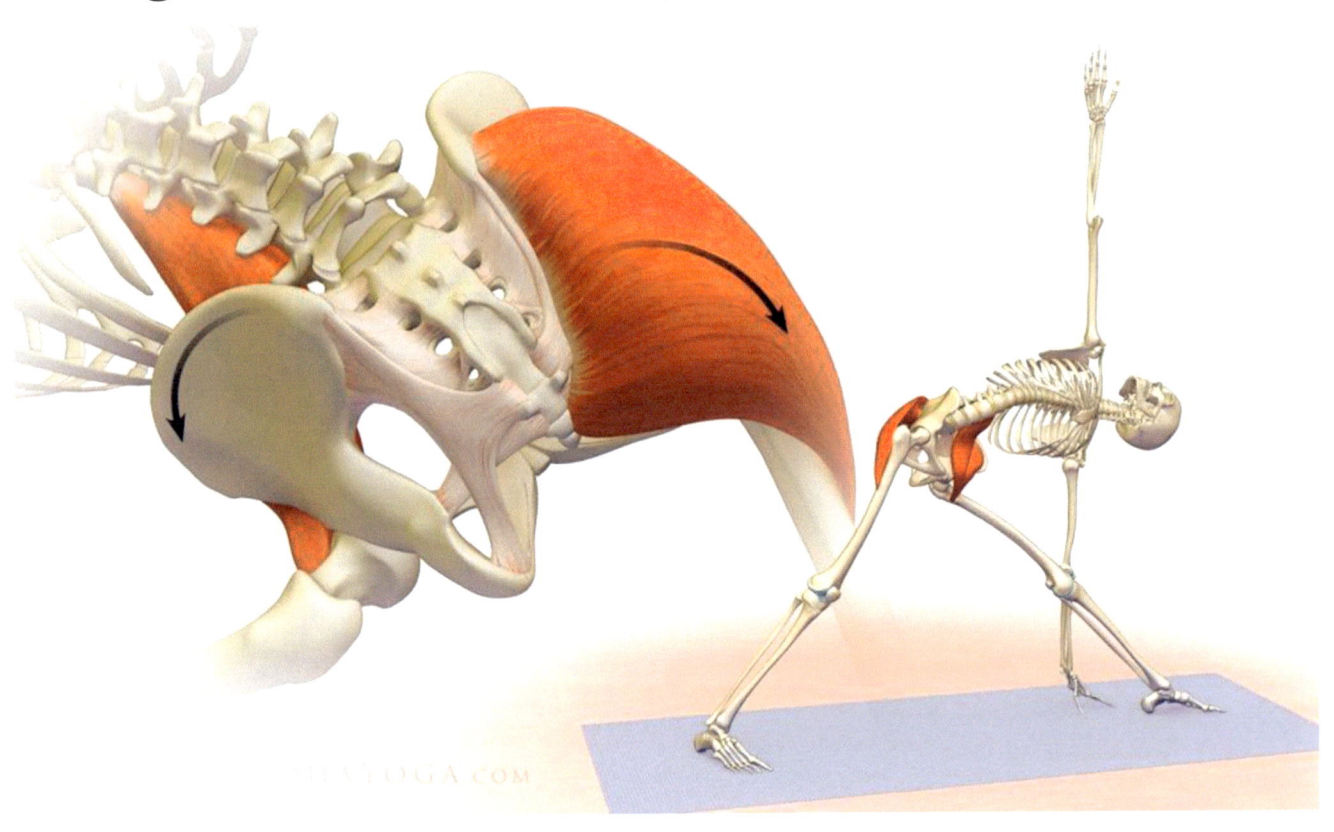

Balance and stabilize your pelvis by contracting your back leg gluteus maximus. Note that the psoas of your forward leg creates a force that tilts your pelvis forward while the glute of the back leg tilts the pelvis back. These two forces act across the strong ligaments of the pelvis to stabilize the entire unit. This is known as "ligamentotaxis". Feel how this action stabilizes your pose from your core.

Figure 3: Balance Contraction with Stretch

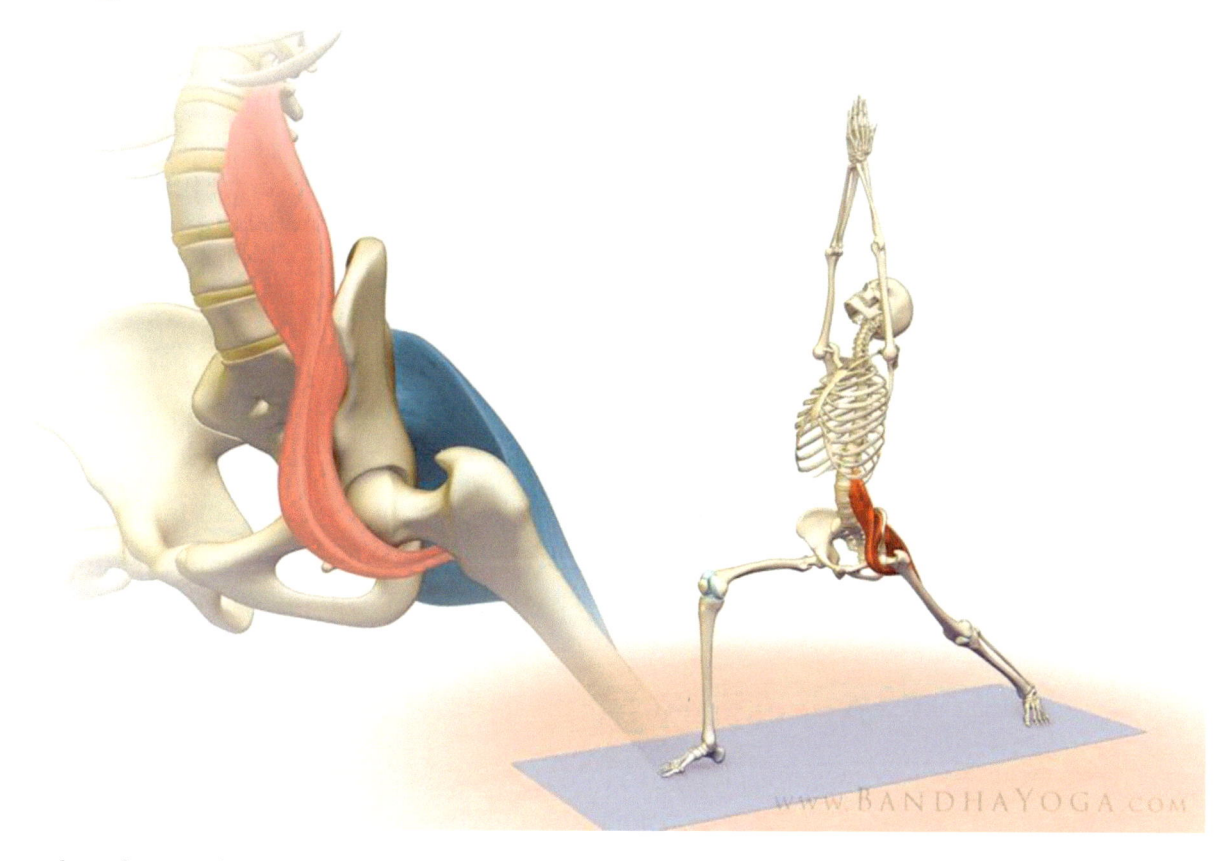

Remember that Hatha Yoga combines opposites—the sun and moon or yin and yang. With this in mind, balance contracting the psoas by stretching it.

Figure 3 illustrates the genius of Hatha Yoga standing poses. While you contract your psoas in the forward leg, you relax and stretch your psoas in the back leg. Thus, each side of the pose balances the other.

Finally, experience "Body Clairvoyance." This refers to the awakened body's ability to anticipate an action and use the most efficient muscles to accomplish it—without thinking about it. The Psoas Awakening Series sequentially activates different parts of the psoas—incrementally and synergistically. When the brain sees a conscious combination of actions like this, it will then automatically use the psoas in unrelated actions. This is analogous to running up a flight of stairs. The first steps are taken consciously, but once we get going, we ascend unconsciously (and rhythmically). The act of typing on a keyboard is another example of this.

Put another way, once we've awakened the dormant psoas muscle, we begin to use it unconsciously in new tasks.

I demonstrate this phenomenon in my workshops by finishing the Psoas Awakening Series with an inversion such as Full Arm Balance. Students regularly report a sensation of rock-solid stability in their pose. This comes from the unconscious brain automatically activating the newly awakened psoas and stabilizing the pelvis. Experience this for yourself by practicing an unrelated asana at the end of the series.

The breath connections

We are more sensitive to the outside world when we are breathing in, whereas the brain tends to tune out when we breathe out. This also aligns with how some extreme sports use breathing. For example, professional marksmen are trained to pull the trigger at the end of exhalation.

In Ujjayi breath you breathe in and out of the nose with the lips sealed – no breath passes the lips. This also serves to build heat in the body. The lips gently close and although the breath is passing through the nostrils, the emphasis is on your throat.

This kind of breathing is done through the nostrils, creating a hissing sound at the back of the throat with both inhalation and exhalation. Simply explained, Ujjayi Pranayama is the process of inhalation and exhalation that is done with both nostrils along with the contraction of the throat muscles.

Accessory Muscles of Breath

The force of the accessory muscles of breath expands the lungs and increases the turbulence of air in the respiratory passageways as a postural muscle. We are generally not conscious of these accessory breath muscles until awakening. Consciously focusing on contracting these muscles brings them under consciousness control with profound effect.

These muscles are found around the shoulders, neck, and upper chest. When they contract, the accessory muscles of inspiration lift the breastbone, upper ribs, and collarbones. This causes the upper part of the chest to rise, making the lungs expand.

Accessory muscles of ventilation include the scalene, the sternocleidomastoid, the pectoralis major, the trapezius, and the external intercostals. Smooth muscle is found in the trachea and in the pulmonary arteries and smaller vessels.

The accessory Muscle of breath straightens the lower back by contacting

The breath connection

Accessory muscles of the breath.
1. Straightening the lower back by contracting the erector spinalis and quadratus. This draws the lower posture rib cage downward.
2. Balance these actions by gently contacting the rectus abnormalities. This draws the lower anterior cage downward and pushes the abdominal organs against the diaphragm, contracting and straightening it.

3. Draw the shoulder blades together by contracting, and this opens the front of the chest.
4. Maintaining this contraction contracts the pectoralis minor and sterno . This lifts and opens the ribcage like elbows.

Exhalation

Access the breath primal force when moving into postures. Gently contract the rectus abdominis, transverse abdominis and intercostal muscles during exhalation. Applying this type of contracting rhythmically connects the conscious and subconscious mind during movement.

Synergy

Train the accessory breathing muscles so that they work synergistically to expand and contract the thorax during movement.

Increase the lung volume during inhalation by contracting the accessory breathing muscles in various combinations. For example, combine the rhomboids with the pectoralis minor or the rectus abdominis with the quadratus lumborum.

Expand the lungs during exhalation by contracting the rectus abdominus, transverse abdominus, and intercostal muscles.

Awakening the accessory breathing muscles is a potent technique that begins with very gentle contraction and progresses slowly and with great care. With any yoga technique, especially breathing, always proceed with caution under the guidance of an instructor.

YOGA ASANAS ABC LEARNING GUIDE

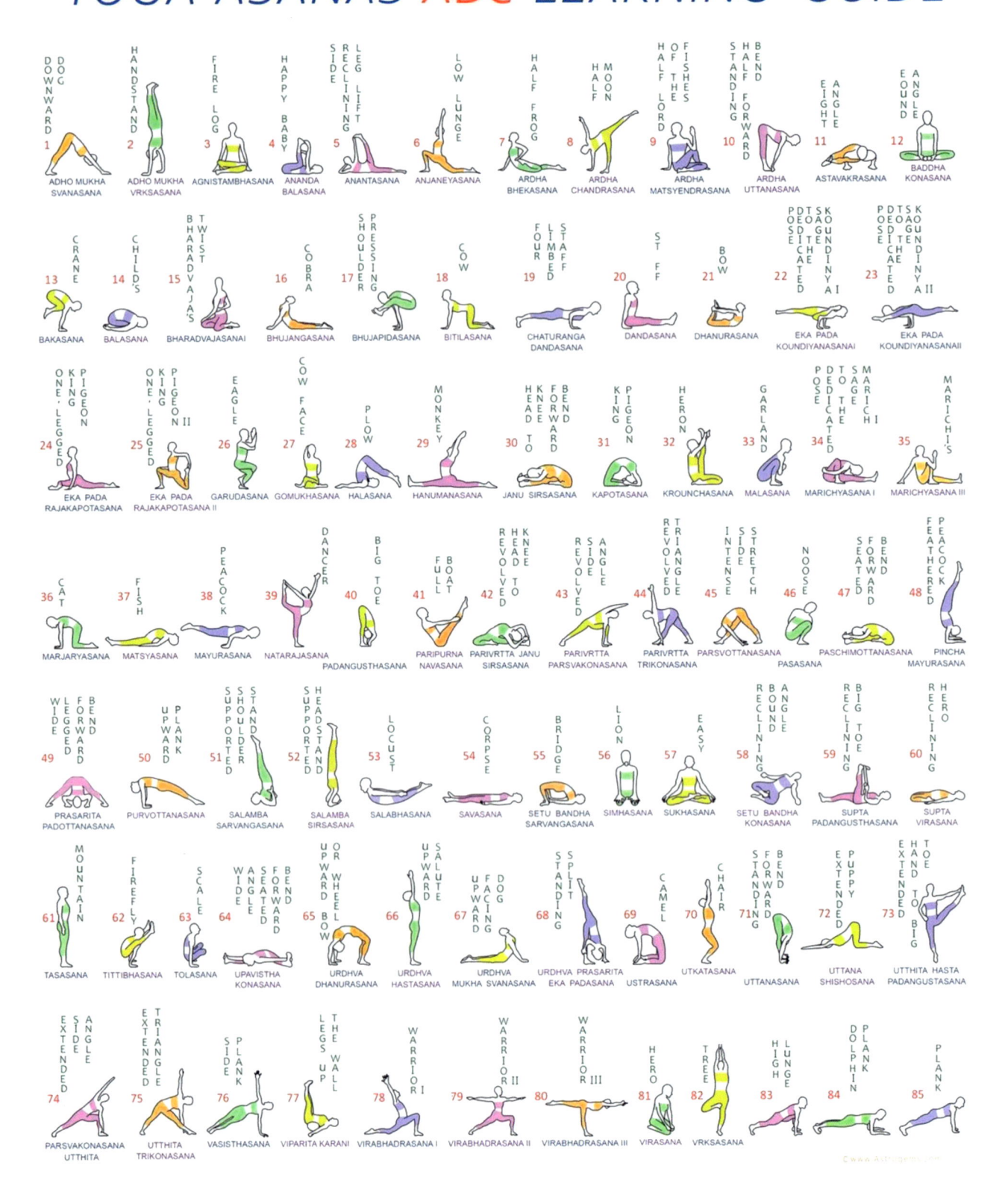

#	Pose	Sanskrit
1	Downward Dog	Adho Mukha Svanasana
2	Handstand	Adho Mukha Vrksasana
3	Fire Log	Agnistambhasana
4	Happy Baby	Ananda Balasana
5	Side Reclining Leg Lift	Anantasana
6	Low Lunge	Anjaneyasana
7	Half Frog	Ardha Bhekasana
8	Half Moon	Ardha Chandrasana
9	Half Lord of the Fishes	Ardha Matsyendrasana
10	Standing Half Forward Bend	Ardha Uttanasana
11	Eight Angle	Astavakrasana
12	Bound Angle	Baddha Konasana
13	Crane	Bakasana
14	Child's	Balasana
15	Bharadvaja's Twist	Bharadvajasana I
16	Cobra	Bhujangasana
17	Shoulder Pressing	Bhujapidasana
18	Cow	Bitilasana
19	Four Limbed Staff	Chaturanga Dandasana
20	Staff	Dandasana
21	Bow	Dhanurasana
22	Pose Dedicated to Koundinya I	Eka Pada Koundiyanasana I
23	Pose Dedicated to Koundinya II	Eka Pada Koundiyanasana II
24	One-Legged King Pigeon	Eka Pada Rajakapotasana
25	One-Legged King Pigeon II	Eka Pada Rajakapotasana II
26	Eagle	Garudasana
27	Cow Face	Gomukhasana
28	Plow	Halasana
29	Monkey	Hanumanasana
30	Head to Knee Forward Bend	Janu Sirsasana
31	King Pigeon	Kapotasana
32	Heron	Krounchasana
33	Garland	Malasana
34	Pose Dedicated to the Sage Marichi	Marichyasana I
35	Marichi's	Marichyasana III
36	Cat	Marjaryasana
37	Fish	Matsyasana
38	Peacock	Mayurasana
39	Dancer	Natarajasana
40	Big Toe	Padangusthasana
41	Full Boat	Paripurna Navasana
42	Revolved Head to Knee	Parivrtta Janu Sirsasana
43	Revolved Side Angle	Parivrtta Parsvakonasana
44	Revolved Triangle	Parivrtta Trikonasana
45	Intense Side Stretch	Parsvottanasana
46	Noose	Pasasana
47	Seated Forward Bend	Paschimottanasana
48	Feathered Peacock	Pincha Mayurasana
49	Wide Legged Forward Bend	Prasarita Padottanasana
50	Upward Plank	Purvottanasana
51	Supported Shoulderstander	Salamba Sarvangasana
52	Supported Headstand	Salamba Sirsasana
53	Locust	Salabhasana
54	Corpse	Savasana
55	Bridge	Setu Bandha Sarvangasana
56	Lion	Simhasana
57	Easy	Sukhasana
58	Reclining Bound Angle	Setu Bandha Konasana
59	Reclining Big Toe	Supta Padangusthasana
60	Reclining Hero	Supta Virasana
61	Mountain	Tasasana
62	Firefly	Tittibhasana
63	Scale	Tolasana
64	Wide Angle Seated Forward Bend	Upavistha Konasana
65	Upward or Wheel Bow	Urdhva Dhanurasana
66	Upward Salute	Urdhva Hastasana
67	Upward Facing Dog	Urdhva Mukha Svanasana
68	Standing Split	Urdhva Prasarita Eka Padasana
69	Camel	Ustrasana
70	Chair	Utkatasana
71	Standing Forward Bend	Uttanasana
72	Extended Puppy	Uttana Shishosana
73	Extended Hand to Big Toe	Utthita Hasta Padangustasana
74	Extended Side Angle	Parsvakonasana Utthita
75	Extended Triangle	Utthita Trikonasana
76	Side Plank	Vasisthasana
77	Legs Up The Wall	Viparita Karani
78	Warrior I	Virabhadrasana I
79	Warrior II	Virabhadrasana II
80	Warrior III	Virabhadrasana III
81	Hero	Virasana
82	Tree	Vrksasana
83	High Lunge	
84	Dolphin Plank	
85	Plank	

Bandhas

Bandha literally means lock, to tighten, to close off and block. There are four main bandhas in the body: Mula Bandha – the root lock, Jalandhara Bandha – the throat lock, Uddiyana Bandha – the lifting of the diaphragm lock.

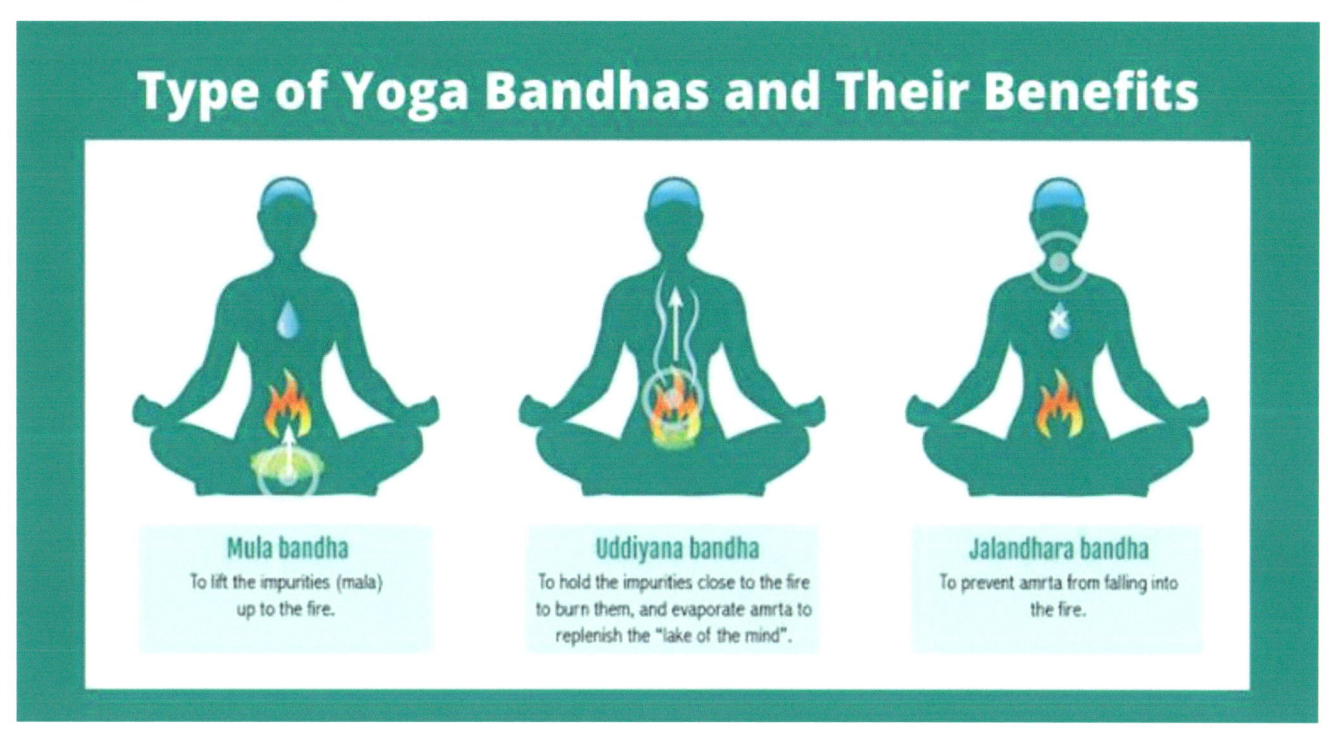

Type of Yoga Bandhas and Their Benefits

Mula bandha
To lift the impurities (mala) up to the fire.

Uddiyana bandha
To hold the impurities close to the fire to burn them, and evaporate amrta to replenish the "lake of the mind".

Jalandhara bandha
To prevent amrta from falling into the fire.

Bandhas are occurring throughout the body. The combination of opposing muscles for these locks stimulates nerve construction and illuminates the chakras.

Mula bandha

Contracts the muscle of the pelvic floor, lifting and toning the organs within the pelvis including the bladder and genitals. The pelvic floor muscles are recruited and awakened by contracting muscles, such as the iliopsoas. This focuses on the mind of the first chakra.

Take, for example, tree pose. Simultaneously contracting other muscle groups, the essential mula bandhas gently squeeze the knees together by contracting the abductors interacting with contraction at the pelvic floor muscles. Pressing the hands together has the same effect this phenomenon shows as recruitment.

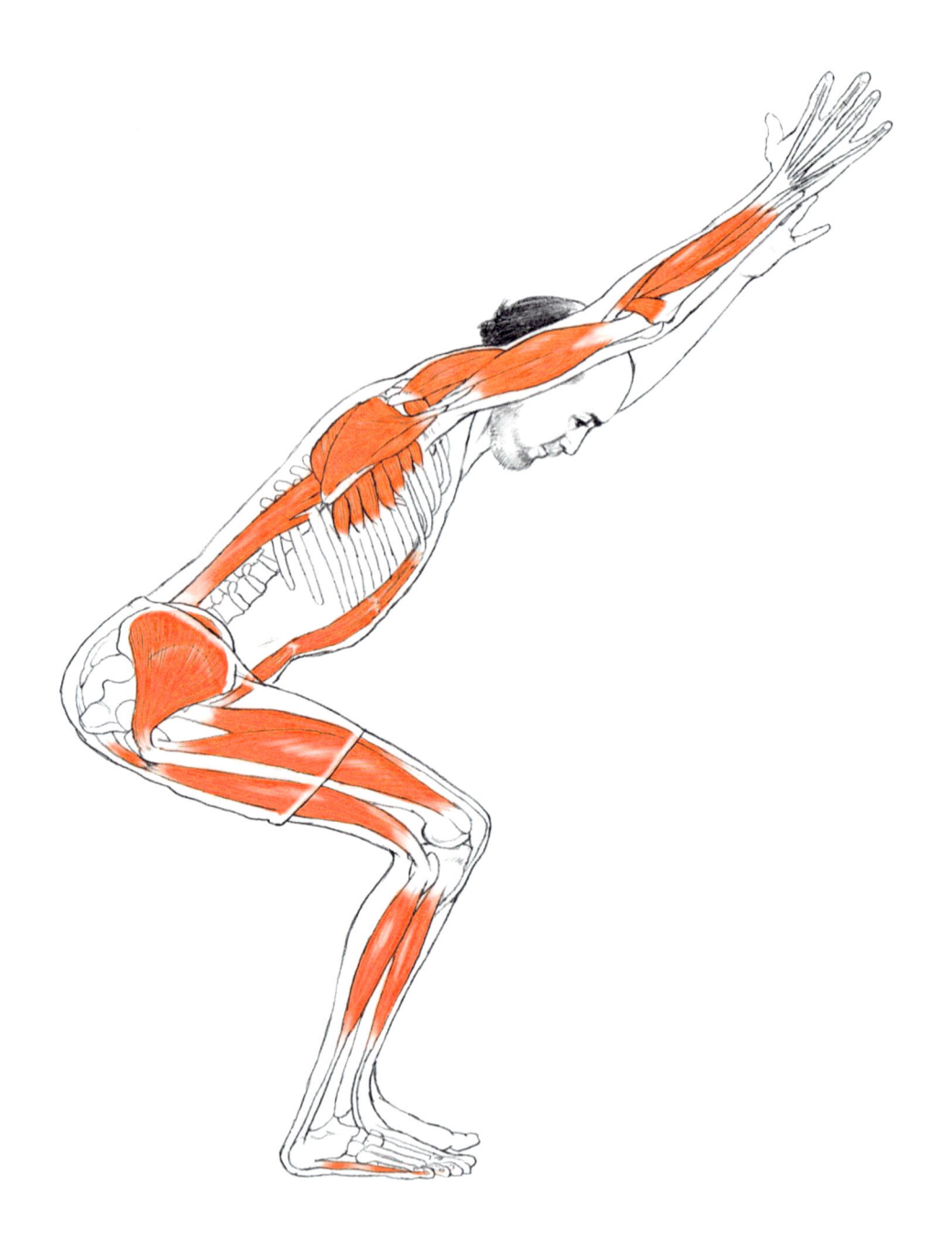

Udyana Bandha

Contracts the upper abdominals in the region approximately two inches below the solar plexus and focuses the mind on the third chakra.

Jotandhara bondha

Contracts the anterior neck muscles, flexing the neck and drawing the chin to the sternum. This focuses the mind on the fifth chakra.

You made it to the end of the course

I am going to attach the test which is open questions.

When you are done with the questions, please submit everything to vyoga4@gmail.com.

I will review and mark your answers, and if you complete the assignment satisfactorily, I will generate your certificate for you via email. If you have any questions, please contact me at vyoga4@gmail.com.

After you receive the certificate, you can apply for Yoga Alliance, and I will approve the course with them from my end.

I hope you enjoyed my course

Yoga is a journey, and life is a journey.

Thanks.

Sincerely, Veronika Patton

QUESTIONS

1. Know the entire sequence from this manual, and please rewrite how you will be teaching it.

2. In your opinion, what is the intention/reason for the sequence?

3. What does the practice of meditation mean to you?

4. Talk about the Bandhas, and the essential elements of each one.

5. Chakra system: There are seven chakras. Please give the name, color, location, and a brief description of each chakra.

6. What are the five elements of assisting a student? Please describe them, such as concentration, intention, confidence, breathing, connection to the earth. Write an example of your direction for each one.

7. Please describe four types of cues with which you can assist your student.

8. Please list the Eight Limbs of Yoga and give a detailed explanation.

9. Describe the importance of energy and how to use it to create a powerful class.

10. What is the most meaningful creation in your life? Is it your work? Family? Yourself?

11. In what areas in your life can you have less reaction and more divine interpretation? For instance, in your relationship, when things get stressful at work, when you are stuck in traffic, when you make a mistake, and so on.

12. Do I give myself enough time to relax and restore myself? How can I carve out more time for relaxation in my life?

13. How much do you believe in yourself, and what role does this play in your everyday life?

14. Do I trust my intuition? If so, or if not, what results does that produce?

15. You will need 20 hours of practice with a teacher. Choose a teacher and ask to observe their class. You will need three different observation classes.

16. In your observation write the intelligence behind the pose, the cues that the teacher used during class, and how it made you feel? What things did you learn each class? You will then submit the three observations to me at Vyoga4u@gmail.com.

17. Film yourself teaching a class and e-mail at me at toVyoga4u@gmail.com.

Congratulations, you've made it to the end of the course. This is an open-question test. When you are done with the questions, please submit your answers to Vyoga4u@gmail.com.

I will review and we'll generate your certificate via e-mail.

Made in the USA
Columbia, SC
24 November 2024